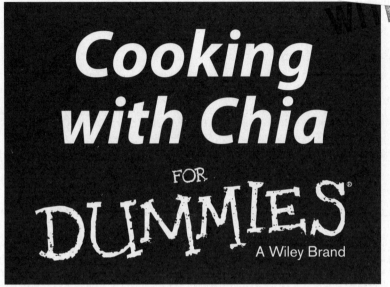

Cooking with Chia

FOR DUMMIES®

A Wiley Brand

by Barrie Rogers and Debbie Dooly

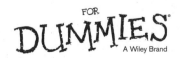

Cooking with Chia For Dummies®

Published by: **John Wiley & Sons, Inc.**, 111 River Street, Hoboken, NJ 07030-5774, www.wiley.com

Copyright © 2014 by John Wiley & Sons, Inc., Hoboken, New Jersey

Published simultaneously in Canada

For general information on our other products and services, please contact our Customer Care Department within the U.S. at 877-762-2974, outside the U.S. at 317-572-3993, or fax 317-572-4002. For technical support, please visit www.wiley.com/techsupport.

Wiley publishes in a variety of print and electronic formats and by print-on-demand. Some material included with standard print versions of this book may not be included in e-books or in print-on-demand. If this book refers to media such as a CD or DVD that is not included in the version you purchased, you may download this material at http://booksupport.wiley.com. For more information about Wiley products, visit www.wiley.com.

Library of Congress Control Number: 2014930401

ISBN 978-1-118-86706-8 (pbk); ISBN 978-1-118-86707-5 (ebk); ISBN 978-1-118-86716-7 (ebk)

Manufactured in the United States of America

10 9 8 7 6 5 4 3 2 1

Contents at a Glance

Recipes at a Glance

Sides

Desserts

Beverages

Table of Contents

Introduction

The typical modern western diet is loaded with processed foods that don't have the nutrients we need to keep up with our fast-paced lives. Because we're not giving our bodies what they need nutritionally, we end up lacking energy in the short term, damaging our vital organs in the long term, and generally not doing ourselves any favors. The good news is, there's a convenient way to boost your nutritional intake and improve your health and well-being. Bring chia seeds into your life!

Chia is a hugely beneficial food that can help you feel more energetic, lose weight, protect your heart, and ease digestive disorders. It does all this with little effort and ticks all the right boxes:

- 100 percent natural
- Gluten free
- Simple to use
- High in essential nutrients

We wrote this book because chia seeds have only become available as a food source in recent years, and we want to give people a comprehensive insight into this wonderful seed so that more people can enjoy its benefits. In this book, we tell you how to find good-quality seeds because not all chia is worth your investment. We also give you over 125 delicious recipes and tips to organize your kitchen that will help get you started.

About This Book

We were thrilled at the prospect of writing a book about chia! We can't stop talking about the fantastic seed that we've benefited from and our families and friends have all benefited from. In this book, we tell you everything you need to know about chia, including its nutritional profile, its benefits, and why it deserves its ranking as a superfood. We provide basic how-to information for using chia and, of course, we share our delicious chia-spiked recipes for you to enjoy.

As with all *For Dummies* books, you don't need to read the book from cover to cover. You can dip into the book to find the information you need. We've organized it so that you can easily jump around and read what interests you today.

Throughout the book, you'll notice text marked with a Technical Stuff icon as well as text in gray boxes, known as sidebars. If this material doesn't interest you, you can safely skip it — you won't lose out on understanding all about chia. On the other hand, if you're as into chia as we are, you'll find this material fascinating and informative.

We follow a few basic conventions in the recipes that you should be aware of:

- ✔ Milk is whole unless otherwise specified.
- ✔ Eggs are large.
- ✔ Pepper is freshly ground black pepper unless otherwise specified.
- ✔ Butter is unsalted.
- ✔ Flour is all-purpose unless otherwise specified.
- ✔ Sugar is granulated unless otherwise noted.
- ✔ All herbs are fresh unless dried herbs are specified.
- ✔ All temperatures are in Fahrenheit. (Refer to the appendix for information about converting temperatures to Celsius.)
- ☺ We use the tomato icon to highlight vegetarian recipes in the Recipes in This Chapter lists, as well as in the Recipes in This Book.

Within this book, you may note that some web addresses break across two lines of text. If you're reading this book in print and want to visit one of these web pages, simply key in the web address exactly as it's noted in the text, pretending as though the line break doesn't exist. If you're reading this as an e-book, you've got it easy — just click the web address to be taken directly to the web page.

Foolish Assumptions

When we sat down to write this book, we made certain assumptions about you:

- ✔ You've at least heard of chia seeds, even if they were only in your novelty potted plants.
- ✔ You may already use chia and know a little bit about it.
- ✔ You may know a great deal about chia and you're simply looking for more ways to use it.
- ✔ You may be interested in healthy foods and want to know how to improve your health through nutrition.
- ✔ You don't want to spend all your time in the kitchen.
- ✔ You want simple but delicious meals that your whole family can enjoy.

Icons Used in This Book

Throughout this book, we use icons to help identify key pieces of information. Here are the different icons we use:

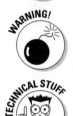

Tips make things easier. We're all about making life a little easier, so if we've found a better way to do something, we mark it with the Tip icon.

The Remember icon give you a heads-up on something important. It may be something you need to take note of or something you need to be aware of before going any further.

Text marked with the Warning icon helps you avoid trouble.

The information next to a Technical Stuff icon can be skipped but it does provide extra information that you may find interesting.

Beyond the Book

In addition to the material in the print or e-book you're reading right now, this product comes with some access-anywhere goodies on the web. Be sure to check out the free Cheat Sheet at www.dummies.com/cheatsheet/cookingwithchia for the top health benefits you can gain from using chia, why athletes use chia, and why chia deserves its reputation as a superfood.

In addition, www.dummies.com/extras/cookingwithchia also contains related articles on everything from how to make chia puddings to how to use chia for endurance.

Where to Go from Here

If you haven't already skipped to the recipes and you want a more detailed explanation of chia, start with Part I, where we give you a good overview of chia and its many health benefits. If you'd rather dive right into the recipes, use the Recipes in This Book and the Table of Contents to find one that sounds good to you. Whether you start with your head or your stomach, you're sure to reap the many rewards that chia has to offer!

Part I
Getting Started with Chia

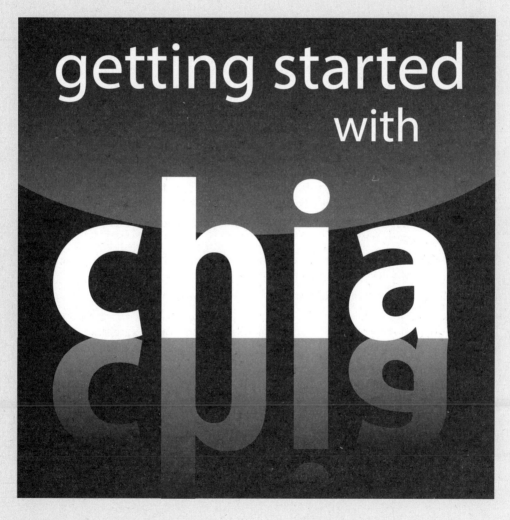

In this part . . .

- ✔ Discover what chia is, who used chia in ancient times, what they used it, for and why it was so important.

- ✔ Compare and contrast chia against flax, its closest competitor.

- ✔ Uncover the nutrients contained in chia and the health benefits you gain from using chia.

- ✔ See how versatile chia is and the endless ways it can be used.

- ✔ Find out how to recognize high-quality chia and how to prepare and use it at home.

Chapter 1

Ch-Ch-Ch-Chia: An Introduction to the Nutrient-Dense Chia Seed

• •

In This Chapter

▶ Finding out what chia is

▶ Delving into the history of chia

▶ Discovering why chia is the ultimate superfood

• •

*G*one are the days when chia was known only because of the Chia Pet. Few people realized the huge nutritional power of those novelty gifts until recently. Chia's popularity has a whole different meaning now, as athletes, nutritionists, and raw food enthusiasts have encouraged its comeback. Chia is a highly nutritious food that can prolong endurance, improve heart health, and encourage good digestion, among many other health benefits that more and more people are discovering every day.

An ancient food that was used by the Aztecs, Mayans, and other cultures, chia has been used for strength, endurance, medicine, currency, and in religious ceremonies as a tribute to gods. It disappeared 500 years ago when the Spanish invaded Central America, but thanks to Dr. Wayne Coates's research efforts, it's back and produced commercially so that people around the world can benefit from these powerful seeds.

Chia is fast becoming the go-to ultimate superfood for athletes, busy moms, people suffering inflammation or digestion problems, and anyone who needs more energy. It packs loads of nutrients into a tiny space and is proving to be easy for all kinds of people to add to their diets and improve their health and well-being.

In this chapter, we fill you in on where chia came from, how it's grown, and why it's making its way to more tables across the United States and around the world. We also compare chia to other seeds. (Spoiler alert: Chia comes out ahead.)

A Simple Seed Brimming with Nutrients

Simple is a great word for chia. The seeds are tiny but powerful, and adding them to your foods is simple. Within these small, black and white seeds are great levels of omega-3 fatty acids, fiber, protein, vitamins, and minerals, and getting these valuable nutrients into your body has never been simpler. The subtle taste of chia means you can add it to anything you already enjoy and it won't affect the flavor whatsoever. This is only one of the many reasons why chia has become so popular as a health food.

Nowadays chia is available in health food stores and supermarkets everywhere. Chia is also becoming an ingredient in more branded foodstuff worldwide. So, you may be asking, "Why this sudden surge in popularity?" Here's why:

- ✔ **Chia is high in omega-3 fatty acids.** Chia is among the highest plant sources of omega-3s in the world. Our bodies need omega-3s for brain function, heart health, and many other biological functions, and most people don't get enough. Chia can help provide more of this essential nutrient.

- ✔ **Chia is high in fiber.** We need fiber in our diets to keep our digestive systems healthy. Chia provides 5 g of fiber in every 15 g serving. It goes a long way toward keeping digestion running smoothly.

- ✔ **Chia is gluten-free.** More people are being diagnosed with gluten intolerance and try to avoid it in their diets. Chia is naturally gluten-free, so it's great for people who have problems with gluten.

- ✔ **Chia is a complete protein.** Chia has all the essential amino acids needed for growth and repair of body cells. This is unusual in a plant. Chia is a great way for vegetarians to get their complete proteins.

- ✔ **Chia is high in vitamins and minerals.** Chia provides high levels of calcium, iron, magnesium, zinc, selenium, folic acid, and many other vitamins and minerals that are needed for various functions in the body.

- ✔ **Chia is 100 percent natural.** Chia provides lots of nutrients, completely naturally. Instead of popping pills, you can eat chia to get nutrition that your body needs.

- ✔ **Chia helps to keep your heart healthy.** The high levels of omega-3 fatty acids and fiber help reduce cholesterol, reduce blood pressure, and protect against cardiovascular disease.

- ✔ **Chia helps prolong endurance.** Chia has long been known for its endurance benefits. The seeds release energy slowly, helping to prolong endurance.

- ✔ **Chia helps balance blood sugar levels.** Chia's *hydrophilic* (water-absorbing) properties help reduce sugar peaks and troughs, helping people to balance their blood sugar levels naturally.

These are just some of the great benefits that chia can provide, the list goes on (see Chapter 2).

A relative to the humble mint leaf

Chia seeds are harvested from a flowering plant called *Salvia hispanica* L. This plant is a member of the mint family, *Lamiaceae*. It's an annual herb that has purple and white flowers that produce the valuable chia seeds. The plant grows to around 3 to 5 feet tall. *Salvia hispanica* L is native to southern Mexico and northern Guatemala, but today it's grown in Argentina, Mexico, Bolivia, and Australia. Trials are happening in a few more countries to test if chia's specific growing conditions can be met elsewhere, so we may see more countries farming chia in the coming years.

Salvia hispanica L loves a sandy soil with good drainage and is grown best in tropical and subtropical conditions. It's a desert plant that is not tolerant of frost. Although the plant needs wet soil to germinate, after that it does well with varying degrees of rainfall. Chia seeds absorb up to ten times their weight in water, which is ideal for a plant that grows in the desert.

The great perk of being related to mint is that insects don't like mint, so they stay away without the use of pesticides. This is fantastic for chia because the seeds are grown in a pesticide-free environment, another bonus for health.

The Endurance Food of Ancient Cultures

Chia seeds have been around a long time. The Aztecs were known to use the seeds, and there is evidence that chia seeds were first used as a food as early as 3500 B.C. The Aztec name for chia was *chian*, which means "oily." Supposedly, when it was translated from Nahuatl, the native language of the Aztecs, it was shortened to *chia*. In another version of the story, chia goes back to the Mayans. The Mayan word *chia* is said to mean "strength." Chia may have been available to the Mayan people, but it was the Aztecs who revered its use and recorded its benefits, so the crop was of utmost importance to the Aztecs. Chia was available to the Aztecs as early as 2600 B.C. Chia went missing for over 500 years, but it's back, and we can all benefit immensely from it.

Chia and the Aztecs

Evidence that the Aztecs used chia appears in codices written 500 years ago. *Codices* were documents written in Nahuatl, the native language of the Aztecs, as well as in Spanish. A lot of them described life at that time and in them, we can see evidence of why chia was used.

Chia was one of four main crops grown by the Aztec cultures. The other three were amaranth, maize (corn), and beans. These four crops served as the basis for the Aztecs' daily diets. Chia seeds were eaten alone, mixed with other grains, ground into flour, used in drinks, and pressed for oil to be used as body and face paints.

Another use for chia was in religious ceremonies. The Aztecs thought so much of chia that they offered the seeds to their gods as worship. They were also paid as tributes to Aztec rulers from conquered nations. One codex describes how 4,410 tons of chia were paid annually to the Aztec Empire.

Chia was valued by the Aztec cultures because of the strength, stamina, and endurance that it provided to their people. A tablespoon of chia was said to sustain Aztec warriors for an entire day! The seeds were also used as medicine and prescribed for wounds, joint pain, sore throats, and sore eyes. Although the Aztecs didn't have the scientific knowledge we do today, they knew that the seeds were highly nutritious. They valued chia as a hugely important crop that could be used for many purposes.

The disappearance of chia

You may wonder why chia disappeared at all if it was such an important part of the Aztec people's daily lives. The answer lies in the conquest of the land by the Spanish. When the Spanish arrived in South America and came upon the Aztecs, they wanted to overtake everything and get rid of the cultures that were there.

Chia disappeared for a few reasons:

- ✔ Chia seeds gave the Aztecs such strength that they thought the seeds gave them almost supernatural powers. Cortez, who led the Spanish invasion, felt that if he got rid of chia, the Aztecs wouldn't last long without it.
- ✔ Because chia was used in religious ceremonies, the friars who came with the Spanish and who wanted to establish their own religions outlawed chia in an attempt to replace the Aztec religions with their own.
- ✔ The Spanish simply liked what they were used to, so they destroyed the chia crops and replaced them with crops that grew well in Spain. Because chia didn't grow in Spain, they assumed it to be of no value.

These reasons together basically ensured that the chia that had been growing in abundance disappeared almost completely. Some crops survived because people fled to the mountains of Central America and continued to grow chia for use within their own communities.

Chia and the Tarahumara Indians

Although the Spanish tried their hardest to abolish chia, it did survive in small clusters thanks to small tribes bringing the seeds to the mountains of Central America after the Spanish had invaded. One of those tribes was the Tarahumara Indians of the Copper Canyon of northern Mexico's Sierra Madre Occidental.

The Tarahumara are a quiet, private tribe, living miles away from each other in caves or small dirt or wooden dwellings. They're known for their long-distance endurance running through narrow footpaths through the canyons.

The Tarahumara were made famous by Christopher McDougall, who wrote about their amazing athletic achievements in his book *Born to Run.* McDougall spent time with some of the Tarahumara and, in his book, writes about the many secrets to their running abilities. In addition to running barefoot, the Tarahumara attribute chia seeds for why they're the world's greatest distance runners. They've always used the seeds to help power their runs, and they often bring pouches of chia with them to munch on along the way.

Chia's resurrection

The resurrection of chia as a hugely beneficial functional food is occurring today as more people continue to discover its benefits and rely on it to provide energy, strength, and endurance again. This is thanks to Dr. Wayne Coates's efforts in bringing the seed back to commercialization so that more people can benefit from it.

Coates led a project in the early 1990s in Argentina that had a mission of looking for alternative crops for farmers. He tested a number of different crops to see if any would have commercial value for farmers in the region. When he tested chia and learned about its great nutritional profile and health benefits, he concentrated on chia and spent years researching the seed and developing the techniques and machinery needed to grow it on a commercial scale. It's thanks to Coates's efforts that we can all benefit from chia today.

Coates still has the goal of bringing chia to as many people as possible at reasonable prices, and he's dedicating his research to this goal. He has written books on chia and continues to educate farmers on how to grow the crop well and ensure that it is cleaned properly before it makes its way to market. He is hugely influential in trying to make sure that only high-quality chia makes it to people's tables. His own brand of high-quality chia is AZChia (www.azchia.com), and he sources and approves chia seeds for our company, Chia bia (www.chiabia.com).

Seeds: They Aren't Just for the Birds

Seeds are making a comeback as a nutrient-dense source of food for everyone, not just the birds. Seeds had a bad reputation for many years, probably because of their high fat content. Thankfully, today we're better educated about the good fats that are essential to good health and are in abundance in many seeds. In addition to good fats, seeds provide large amounts of protein, complex carbohydrates, fiber, vitamins, and minerals.

Throughout history, seeds have been used as an important nutrient source by many cultures — and rightly so. They provide loads of energy and go a long way toward providing the trace minerals that are often absent in western diets. Seeds also help protect against disease because they provide the phytochemicals that help fight illness.

Not only do seeds provide vegetarians and vegans with a great source of protein, but they offer great nutrition in tiny bundles to everyone, regardless of what kind of diet you like to enjoy. The birds always knew that seeds were a good choice of food, and chia seeds are tops when it comes to the choice of seeds out there.

Comparing common seeds

Most seeds are a great nutrient-dense food, but how does chia compare nutritionally to some of the other seeds available? The most common seeds that people add to foods are sunflower seeds, pumpkin seeds, and flaxseeds. Table 1-1 offers a comparison of these and other common seeds.

Table 1-1	How Chia Seeds Stacks Up to Other Seeds (Per 100 g)			
	Fiber	*Antioxidants*	*Protein*	*Omega-3 Fatty Acids*
Chia seeds	34.4 g	6,530 μ mol	16.54 g	17.8 g
Flaxseeds	27.3 g	Trace	18.3 g	22.8 g
Hemp seeds	12.0 g	Trace	25.0 g	7.0 g
Sunflower seeds	11.1 g	Trace	19.3 g	0.069 g
Pumpkin seeds	6.5 g	Trace	29.8 g	0.11 g
Sesame seeds	11.8 g	Trace	17.7 g	0.4 g

Source: U.S. Department of Agriculture, National Nutrient Database for Standard Reference

As you can see, chia is very high in omega-3 fatty acids, but where it really surpasses all other seeds is its level of antioxidants. Chia is also higher in fiber than any of the other seeds. So, when compared to other seeds, chia really is the nutritional winner. The only seed that is comparable in nutrient value is flax, but chia has other properties that flax just can't compete with (see the nearby sidebar, "Chia versus flax: Which wins?").

This table only measures the nutrient value of seeds. We discuss chia's other properties in the next section.

Chia: A unique seed with special properties

No other seed has as many great properties in one tiny bundle as chia does. Here are the unique properties that set chia apart from any other seeds on the market:

- **Hydrophilic:** Chia can absorb up to ten times its weight in water, which is a great property to have when it comes to weight loss. The water it absorbs fills your stomach and helps you feel fuller longer.

- **Subtle taste:** Because chia has little or no taste, it can be added to foods without affecting the flavor.

- **Slow energy release:** The energy that chia provides is released slowly because a physical barrier is formed to slow the conversion of carbohydrates to sugars. This is fantastic for people who want to balance blood sugar levels, such as those who have diabetes.

- **No need to grind:** Chia has a soft outer shell, so your body can break it down easily and absorb the nutrients inside. You don't need to grind chia seeds before eating them.

- **Long shelf life:** Once harvested, chia has a shelf life of up to five years.

Chia versus flax: Which wins?

Flaxseeds are great seeds to add to your diet — they're very high in the all-important omega-3s that we all need more of and chia is often compared to flax because it has similar amounts of omega 3 and some other nutrients. But we think chia has the edge. Here's why:

- Chia is full of antioxidants where flax has only trace levels of antioxidants (refer to Table 1-1).

- Chia beats flax in terms of fiber, calcium, and selenium. Flax beats chia in terms of magnesium and potassium.

- Chia has less fat and fewer calories than flax.

- Chia is hydrophilic, and flax is not.

- Chia is bioavailable, and flax is not. You don't need to grind chia seeds — your body is capable of digesting its soft shell and absorbing the nutrients. Flax has a hard, indigestible shell and it needs to be ground down before you eat it in order for your body to be able to absorb the nutrients.

- Chia has a longer shelf life than flax. Chia's shelf life is up to five years after it's harvested. Flax has a shelf life of a maximum of two years after it's harvested, but usually flax is ground to release its nutrients, and ground flaxseeds typically last around 6 to 16 weeks if stored correctly.

- Chia is pretty much taste-free, which means you can add it to a variety of foods and recipes to boost the nutrient profile. Flax has a distinctive taste that some people just don't like, and because it has a taste, you can't add it to other recipes without altering the taste.

All in all, we believe chia is the hands-down winner when it comes to packing a nutritional punch. No wonder the tiny seed is replacing flax in many people's diets!

Chapter 2

Getting Your Nutritional Facts Right: The Tiny Seed with a Mighty Punch

....

In This Chapter

▶ Identifying the nutrients contained in chia

▶ Discovering the different fatty acids

▶ Realizing the importance of fiber in the diet

▶ Gaining from the power of protein and antioxidants

▶ Avoiding modern-day nutritional pitfalls

....

*E*ating a nutrient-packed diet is the most important thing you can do for your body, and chia provides many of the nutrients you need to stay healthy. In fact, chia is so chock-full of nutrients that it may even be possible to live on chia and water alone and satisfy all your nutritional needs. Of course, you may find that diet a bit boring, and your friends may stop accepting your dinner invitations. The good news is, you don't have to live off chia to reap the many health benefits this little seed has to offer. Instead, because chia is almost tasteless, you can add it to whatever you already enjoy eating, boosting your meal's nutrients.

In this chapter, we tell you what to look for when reading food labels, describe the nutrients your body requires, and explain how chia can provide your body with these nutrients that are so essential for good health.

The Nutritional Profile of Chia

Good nutrition is continuing to be recognized around the world as the key to good health as more people are using different nutrients to help combat certain diseases and improve different aspects of their health and well-being. Chia is made up of important nutrients that are essential for good health.

Navigating chia food labels

To understand what nutrients are in chia and products containing chia, your first stop should be the Nutrition Facts label (shown in Figure 2-1). This label tells you everything from the suggested serving size to the ingredients to how much of the various nutrients the food contains. When you understand exactly how to read a Nutrition Facts label and what to look for, you'll be on your way to easily tracking your daily intake.

The Nutrition Facts label lists the following:

- ✔ **Serving size:** How much of the food you'll typically eat in one sitting. A typical serving size of chia is 15 g, which is approximately 2 tablespoons of seeds.

    We recommend that you get one serving of chia per day.

- ✔ **Servings per container:** How many servings you get in the bag, box, carton, or container. The servings per container is handy when you're comparing different size bags of chia seeds.

- ✔ **Calories:** The number of calories in one serving. A 15 g serving of chia seeds is approximately 69 calories. When it comes to daily caloric intake (around 2,000 calories per day), that's not much! That means you can add one serving of chia seeds to your day without loosening your belt.

- ✔ **Fat:** Fats have gotten a bad rep, but not all fats are bad for you — in fact, you need fat your diet. The Nutrition Facts label tells you the total amount of fat in the food, as well as the amount of saturated fat and trans fat (the bad kinds). Some labels also tell you the amount of polyunsaturated and monounsaturated fats (the good kinds). Chia has no trans fat and less than 0.5 g of saturated fat per serving, which is a tiny amount.

    You don't need to worry about the fats contained in chia — they're almost entirely good fats that your body needs.

- ✔ **Cholesterol:** High cholesterol is a risk factor for coronary heart disease, which is why people are always trying to reduce their cholesterol levels. You have nothing to worry about when it comes to chia, because it contains no cholesterol. In fact, it actually helps in the fight to reduce blood cholesterol levels!

- ✔ **Sodium:** Although your body needs sodium, the typical modern diet has far too much sodium. Consuming too much sodium can increase blood pressure and lead to heart complications, so limiting your sodium intake is a good idea. The good news is, chia has no sodium, so you can be confident you're not adding to your sodium intake when you consume chia.

- ✔ **Carbohydrate:** Carbohydrates provide the body with energy, but not all carbohydrates are created equal. Refined carbohydrates, such as the type found in white breads, cereals, or pasta, are not the healthiest carbohydrates; they should be eaten only in small amounts. Lucky for you, chia is not a refined carbohydrate so you don't have to worry about consuming it.

Nutrition Facts

Serving Size 2 Tablespoons (15g)
Servings Per Container: 26

Amount Per Serving

Calories 69   Calories from Fat 21

% Daily Value*

Total Fat 4.6g	**7**%
Saturated Fat 0.5g	**3**%
Trans Fat 0g	
Cholesterol 0mg	**0**%
Sodium 0mg	**0**%
Total Carbohydrate 5g	**2**%
Dietary Fiber 5g	**20**%
Sugars 0g	
Protein 3.1g	**6**%

Vitamin A	1%
Vitamin C	3%
Calcium	9%
Iron	6%
Magnesium	13%

*Percent Daily Values are based on a 2,000 calorie diet. Your Daily Values may be higher or lower depending on your calorie needs:

	Calories:	2,000	2,500
Total Fat	Less than	65g	80g
Saturated Fat	Less than	20g	25g
Cholesterol	Less than	300mg	300mg
Sodium	Less than	2,400mg	2,400mg
Total Carbohydrate		300g	375g
Dietary Fiber		25g	30g

Figure 2-1: A typical Nutrition Facts label for chia seeds.

© John Wiley & Sons, Inc.

Under the amount of total carbohydrate, you'll see the following:

- **Dietary fiber:** Fiber is very powerful — it helps decrease the appetite and slows the conversion of carbohydrates to sugars, giving you a slow release of energy. Chia contains 5 g of fiber per serving, but what's even better is that chia contains both soluble *and* insoluble fiber; the latter is needed for good digestive health. (See the later section "The Fiber Boost Found in Chia" for more on fiber.)

- **Sugars:** Added sugar is proving to be detrimental to health and is thought to be one of the leading causes of the rising rates of obesity worldwide. Chia contains no sugar, so you don't need to worry about adding sugar to your diet with chia.

  Be careful when purchasing food products containing chia. Although there are no added sugars in chia seeds alone, the products containing chia may have plenty added sugars. Read the label to know what you're getting.

✔ **Protein:** Chia contains all nine essential amino acids, making it a complete high-quality protein (see the later section "Chia: A Complete Protein," for more on amino acids). Protein is a very important factor when assessing the nutritional profile of chia. Each serving has 3.1 g of this high-quality meat-free protein. Because of how much protein it has, chia can serve as an alternative to soy in vegetarian diets.

At the bottom of the food label, you see a list of some vitamins and minerals, and the Percent Daily Values that the food contains. So, for example, if the label lists vitamin A and says it has 10 percent, that means that one serving of the food gives you 10 percent of the vitamin A you should get every day.

Chia contains many vitamins and minerals. Here's why vitamins and minerals are important for your health and info on some of the vitamins and minerals chia contains:

✔ **Vitamins:** Vitamins are essential for normal growth and body functions. You have to ingest them (through food or supplements) because the body can't produce enough of them on its own.

The vitamins that are listed on the chia food label (refer to Figure 2-1) are

- **Vitamin A:** Vitamin A is important for growth and development and for the maintenance of the immune system. It's also important for good vision. One 15 g serving of chia provides 1.08 percent of the vitamin A you need daily.

- **Vitamin C:** Vitamin C supports normal growth and development and helps your body absorb iron. One 15 g serving of chia provides you with 2.7 percent of the vitamin C you need every day.

✔ **Minerals:** Minerals work alongside other nutrients to help your body function properly and stay healthy. Similar to vitamins, you need to ingest them (through food or supplements). Chia contains many minerals, but only calcium, iron, and magnesium are listed on the Nutrition Facts label (see the next section for what's not on the label).

- **Calcium:** Calcium is needed for bone development and is essential for maintaining strong bones and teeth. It also prevents *osteoporosis* (a disease in which bones become more brittle and likely to break), which affects many people, particularly women, as they age. One 15 g serving of chia provides 8.5 percent of the calcium you need every day.

- **Iron:** Your body needs iron for the delivery of oxygen to cells. Lack of iron can result in fatigue and decreased immunity. One 15 g serving of chia provides 5.8 percent of the iron you need daily.

- **Magnesium:** Magnesium is needed for almost all body functions, from energy production and enzyme activation to the regulation of other nutrient levels. Teeth, bones, the heart, kidneys, and muscles all need magnesium to function. One 15 g serving of chia provides 12.6 percent of the magnesium you need every day.

Recognizing what's not on the label

Food labels are great, but they can't possibly tell you everything. There is so much more to chia than can fit on a typical food label! The vitamins and minerals found in chia that are *not* listed on the label provide great health benefits to your body and are well worth noting.

Here are the most common and important vitamins and minerals that chia offers but that may not be listed on the Nutrition Facts label:

- ✔ **Vitamin B1 (thiamin):** Thiamin is one of eight B vitamins, all of which help the body convert food into energy. These B vitamins (often referred to as the *vitamin B complex*) are needed for healthy skin, hair, eyes, and liver. They also help the nervous system function properly and are needed for good brain function. One 15 g serving of chia contains 8.4 percent of the vitamin B1 you need every day.

- ✔ **Vitamin B3 (niacin):** Niacin is another of the eight B vitamins. It helps improve circulation. One 15 g serving of chia contains 8.9 percent of the vitamin B3 you need daily.

- ✔ **Folate (folic acid):** Folate is essential for numerous bodily functions, such as synthesizing and repairing DNA. It's especially important in aiding rapid cell division and growth, such as infancy and pregnancy. One 15 g serving of chia provides 1.8 percent of the folate you need every day.

- ✔ **Selenium:** Selenium acts as an antioxidant in the body and helps prevent the buildup of free radicals in the blood that can damage cells. It's also known to benefit the thyroid and aid the immune system. One 15 g serving of chia provides 11.8 percent of the selenium you need daily.

Who says? Looking at Recommended Dietary Allowances

People everywhere — from nutritionists and dietitians to doctors and athletes — have differing opinions on how much of everything we should be consuming every day. This, combined with the fact that all individual nutritional needs vary, leads to confusion. A young, active boy will have very different nutritional needs than an older woman leading a more sedentary lifestyle. This makes it extremely difficult to put a figure on how much of any particular nutrient is needed on a daily basis.

However, government agencies around the world have tried to do just that. They've come up with Recommended Dietary Allowances (RDAs), which, according to the Office of Dietary Supplements at the National Institutes of Health are the "average daily level of intake sufficient to meet the nutrient requirements of nearly all healthy people." The RDAs for nutrients vary from one country to the next, so any time we state an RDA in this book, we're referring to the U.S. Department of Agriculture (USDA) RDAs. We're also referring to the RDAs for adults, unless we note otherwise.

✔ **Zinc:** Zinc is best known for its role in maintaining ideal hormone levels. It can help balance blood sugar levels and help strengthen the immune system. One 15 g serving of chia provides 5.7 percent of the zinc you need every day.

Chia and Its Fatty Acids

Fat has been the victim of some bad press the last few decades. But what the news articles often fail to mention is that there are different kinds of fat, some of which are good for you! The general public didn't know the differences between these types of fat, so all fats got a bad name and people thought they needed to drop fat from their diets completely. Dropping fats completely from your diet would be detrimental to your health — certain fats are needed for brain and hormone function and keeping your heart healthy. The fatty acids contained in chia seeds are mostly these essential fatty acids that are required for good health.

In this section, we walk you through the good fats you need and tell you where to find them.

What omega-3 fatty acids are and where you can find them

Omega-3 fatty acids help build new cells and regulate various processes of the body. Our bodies can't make omega-3s, so we need to get them from food or supplements. In addition to boosting heart health by lowering cholesterol and reducing blood pressure, omega-3s are key to healthy skin, hair, and nails. Everything from depression and attention deficit hyperactivity disorder (ADHD) to increases in chronic diseases and lack of concentration has been blamed on the lack of omega-3s in the modern diet. This is why so many governments, dietitians, and nutritionists are recommending that people increase their intake of omega-3s.

Numerous studies into the effects of omega-3s on the body — for example, improvements in heart health and circulation, reduction in inflammation, and improved brain function — have led to this increase in demand for omega-3s as more people continue to realize its benefits. Chia is the best plant-based source of omega-3s in the world, making it a fantastic way to get enough of this all-important nutrient.

There are a variety of different types of omega-3 fatty acids, but three you should know about are

✔ Alpha-linolenic acid (ALA)

✔ Docosahexaenoic (DHA)

✔ Eicosapentaenoic (EPA)

The omega-3s found in fish and fish oil are DHA and EPA. Although fish can be a healthy part of your diet, the omega-3s found in fish and fish oil aren't without problems:

✔ If the fish you eat is farmed instead of wild, it doesn't contain omega-3s naturally — the fish has to be fed omega-3 supplements in order to contain omega-3s, which means you're better off opting for wild fish than farmed.

✔ Not all fish oils are good sources of DHA and EPA. Even though you get good levels of these omega-3s, you may be getting more than you bargained for. Fish that has been primarily in polluted waters can contain pollutants that are bad for health, so fish oil capsules may not be the best option for getting omega-3s.

✔ In recent years, there has been some concern about the sustainability of fish that are harvested for omega-3 fish oil. Overfishing worldwide has become a cause for concern — certain species of fish that are used for fish oil production are becoming endangered. Plant-based omega-3s are a sustainable source for human consumption.

The omega-3 fatty acid found in chia seeds is ALA, which is derived from plants and, when eaten, converted to DHA and EPA. Your body will convert the ALA to as much DHA and EPA as it needs and excrete the rest, so you don't have to worry about eating too much ALA.

Omega-6 and the omega-3–to–omega-6 ratio

Omega-6 is another essential fatty acid that the body can't produce. It's found in many vegetable oils and animal fats. In the typical modern diet, people consume plenty of omega-6s. This makes it easy to get your fill of omega-6s. The problem is that we eat too much of omega-6 and not nearly enough of omega-3.

Back when modern people were evolving from hunter/gatherers, the ratio of omega-3 to omega-6 fatty acids that they typically ate was 1:1. These days, people eat an average of 1:20 (omega-3 to omega-6). This imbalance increases the risk of coronary heart disease and other modern-day chronic diseases.

Consuming enough omega-3s can help restore the proper balance. The ratio of omega-3s to omega-6s in chia is 3:1, helping you restore balance in your diet.

The Fiber Boost Found in Chia

Fiber (or what your grandma may have referred to as "roughage") is the part of food that your body can't digest. Even though the body can't digest it, fiber provides many health benefits and is essential for a healthy diet. Unlike fats, proteins, or carbohydrates, which your body breaks down and absorbs, fiber isn't digested by your body — it passes through the digestive system relatively intact. Fiber is mainly found in fruits, vegetable, legumes, and whole grains, but chia is also a fantastic source of fiber, providing 5 g of fiber per 15 g serving of chia. This equates to 20 percent of the fiber you need in a day. That's a lot of fiber for such a small portion of food with little calories!

Why fiber matters

Most people know that we need fiber in the diet, but not everyone knows why. Here's what fiber does for you:

- ✔ **Helps you maintain a healthy weight:** Because chia is high in fiber, it helps to make you feel fuller longer, reducing cravings for unhealthy foods. This can help maintain a healthy body weight.

Soluble versus insoluble fiber

There are different types of fiber:

✔ **Soluble:** Soluble fiber mixes well with water, swells, and forms a gel-like substance that slows digestion. It also slows the rate of glucose absorption, thereby reducing cholesterol absorption. Soluble fiber is what makes you feel fuller longer, helping you eat less. Soluble fiber is also great for balancing blood sugar levels.

✔ **Insoluble:** Insoluble fiber does not mix with water. It provides bulk to the diet and essentially leaves the body much like it enters the body, helping to keep digestion running smoothly and preventing constipation along the way.

Both soluble and insoluble fiber are important for digestive health. Chia has a great mix of both fibers, so you can be sure you're getting the right fiber needed for good digestive health.

✔ **Reduces constipation:** Dietary fiber adds weight and bulk to stools and softens it, making it easier to pass and decreasing the chance of constipation.

TIP

When you're increasing your fiber intake, make sure you're drinking plenty of water. Otherwise, you could end up getting constipated — the opposite of the effect you're looking for. Aim for drinking at least eight 8-ounce glasses of water per day.

✔ **Lowers cholesterol levels:** Soluble fiber (see the nearby sidebar) may help lower total blood cholesterol levels by reducing LDL (bad) cholesterol. Studies have revealed that viscous fibers, like the soluble fiber in chia, are most effective in reducing blood cholesterol levels.

✔ **Reduces the risk of cardiovascular disease:** Fiber is proving to have other heart-healthy benefits such as reduced blood pressure and inflammation, which help in the fight against cardiovascular disease.

✔ **Reduces the risk of hemorrhoids:** A high-fiber diet lowers the risk of developing hemorrhoids. And that's something we can all get behind (no pun intended).

✔ **Controls blood sugar levels:** The soluble fiber found in chia slows the absorption of sugar, helping to balance blood sugar levels. This is great for people with diabetes because it provides a natural way to help balance blood sugar levels.

How much fiber is enough

When it comes to fiber, the experts always say to eat more. But how much more often isn't clear. Depending on your age and gender, you should try to consume 20 g to 38 g of dietary fiber per day. (Fiber intake can be reduced a little for children.) Table 2-1 breaks it down for you.

Table 2-1	How Much Fiber Is Enough	
Gender	Age 50 or Younger	Over Age 50
Male	38 g	30 g
Female	25 g	21 g

Most Americans eat less than 15 g of fiber a day, which is why so many Americans suffer from diseases such as irritable bowel syndrome (IBS).

Each 15 g serving of chia provides 5 g of fiber, which gets you well on your way to reaching your goal. You can also increase your fiber intake by eating more fruits, vegetables, beans, lentils, and whole grains.

Chia: The Power of a Complete Protein

Protein is another important nutrient that is essential for building, maintaining, and replacing the cells in your body, as well as making enzymes, hormones, and other body chemicals. You need to take in good-quality proteins to keep up with this manufacture of body tissue. The most common sources of protein are meat, fish, eggs, dairy, nuts, and seeds. Chia is a great source of protein — not only is chia made up of 21 percent protein, but it's a high-quality complete protein that our bodies crave.

Chia is a complete protein because it contains all nine essential amino acids that are needed for building complete cells. Amino acids are the building blocks of life. Scientists have identified 22 amino acids as important to human health, but our bodies can make only 13 of these, which means we need to get the remaining 9 from our foods. This is why these nine amino acids are called *essential amino acids*. Often, plant proteins are missing some of these essential amino acids, so our bodies need to get them from other sources — but not with chia! Chia is one of the few non-meat, non-dairy foods that has all nine essential amino acids.

Chia is a great food for anyone following a plant-based diet because it provides the body with the complete proteins that it needs to build and maintain body tissues without the saturated fats that come with eating meats. So, not only is chia a fantastic source of protein for vegetarians and vegans, but it's a great source of protein for everyone!

The Antioxidants That Give Chia the Edge

Chia is chock-full of naturally occurring antioxidants that really give it the edge when it comes to packing nutrients into small spaces. Antioxidants protect delicate essential fatty acids from oxidation. Unlike other plant sources of omega-3s, such as flaxseeds, chia doesn't require added artificial antioxidants in order to remain fresh. So, chia seeds remain fresh longer and don't require refrigeration, thanks to their abundance of natural antioxidants.

One measure that has been developed to describe overall antioxidant capacity of foods is called oxygen radical absorbance capacity (ORAC). Chia seeds have a relatively high ORAC value, ranging from 60 to 80 micromoles. The antioxidants found in chia include flavonoids (quercetin, kaempferol, and myricetin) and the phenolic acids (chlorogenic and caffeic acid). These antioxidants have significant value to human health — they've been shown to reduce oxidative stress caused by free radicals in the body, thus helping to prevent the onset of common degenerative diseases.

Avoiding the Bad Stuff: Processed Foods and Hidden Sugar

Eating a healthy diet that's high in fiber, good fats, quality proteins, and vitamins and minerals, but low in sugar, salt, and saturated fats can do wonders for your health, helping you maintain a healthy weight, keeping your heart and digestion healthy, and keeping you full of energy. However, when you look at what's available to buy on our supermarket shelves (processed foods and foods high in hidden sugars), it becomes very difficult to strike a healthy balance. If you can learn to avoid these two dangers, you'll be well on your way to a balanced diet.

The onslaught of processed foods

Today's consumers are looking for convenient and cheap foods with a long shelf life. The food industry meets these consumer demands by processing foods. A *processed food* is a food that has been changed from its natural state either by adding something to it (such as additives or preservatives) or by doing something to it (such as freezing, dehydrating, or applying heat treatments). Processing a food alters the natural healthy enzymes, fatty acids, vitamins, and minerals. Processed foods can cause health problems if consumed in large quantities.

Some common examples of processed foods are white wheat flour, artificial sweeteners, margarine, fast foods, soft drinks, packaged cakes, cookies, processed meat, frozen dinners, soy products, refined sugars . . . the list is practically endless. You may not even realize that some of the foods you eat are processed, so be sure to read food labels — look out for ingredients that you find difficult to pronounce. Avoid anything with a long list of unrecognizable ingredients. Also, look out for the sugar content on the food label and avoid foods that are very high in sugar.

Not all processed foods are bad. In some cases, food processing is helpful. For example, freezing vegetables when they're picked helps maintain their high nutritional values and can be both beneficial and convenient.

Foods such as pastured, grass-fed meats, eggs, and poultry; fresh vegetables and fruits; wild-caught seafood; and raw nuts and seeds support your body. Stick with these types of foods for the majority of your meals, and you'll go a long way toward avoiding the health problems associated with processed junk foods.

Hidden sugars: They're everywhere

To understand hidden sugars, you need to understand carbohydrates. Carbohydrates are an essential source of energy for our bodies, but there are both good carbs and bad carbs.

Good carbs are foods that are in their natural state and haven't been processed. These carbs are generally high in fiber, will give you energy over a longer period of time and keep you feeling full. Examples of good carbs are seeds, nuts, vegetables, and whole-grain breads, cereals, and pastas.

Bad carbs are foods that have been refined and processed; they're high in calories and generally have no nutritional value. People who eat too many bad carbs are at greater risk of developing diabetes, heart disease, and obesity. Bad carbs give you a temporary spike in energy, but your energy levels fall off sharply, making you crave more bad carbs. And the cycle continues. . . .

The majority of bad carbs are refined sugars and are used in processed foods. When you read a food label, look at the grams of carbohydrates and the grams of sugar. The further apart these numbers, the better. An example of a bad carb would be a chocolate bar, which could have 40 g of carbs and 40 g of sugar per serving. An example of a good carbohydrate would be whole-grain pasta, which could have 45 g of carbs and 2.6 g of sugar per serving — a reasonable amount.

Keep the gap between carbs and sugars as far apart as possible.

Chapter 3

Unleashing the Disease-Fighting Power of Chia

In This Chapter

▶ Understanding chia's role in brain function

▶ Seeing how chia can help heal your body

*W*hen it comes to keeping your mind and body healthy, you are what you eat. In this chapter, we look at how the nutrients in chia can help bring balance back to your diet and, therefore, help with many of the diseases we face today, including diabetes, heart disease, high cholesterol, high blood pressure, and even Alzheimer's disease and depression.

This chapter is all about how chia can provide your body with the tools it needs to keep your mind and body healthy and enable them to fight disease.

The Mind: Feeding Your Brain

Eating well is just as important for your mental health as it is for your physical health. The brain needs nutrients to function just like the rest of your body does. If you eat the wrong foods, or too much food, you can gain weight and cause other health problems that you may be able to see physically, but a bad diet is detrimental to what goes on in the brain, too. When you don't feed your brain with the nutrients it needs, it can't function well. The brain needs fat, protein, and carbohydrate to function properly, and it also needs antioxidants to defend itself from harm:

✔ **Fat:** Two-thirds of the brain is made up of fat, and the brain needs healthy fatty acids to produce brain cells. These fatty acids form the membrane surrounding your brain cells — fuel passes in and waste passes out. Omega-3 alpha-linolenic acid (ALA) and omega-6 fatty acids are essential fatty acids — you need to consume them because your body can't make them. The body uses ALA and omega-6 fatty acids to make DHA fatty acids in the brain, and DHA is essential for the brain to function.

If you don't consume essential fatty acids through food and/or supplements, you aren't giving your brain the nutrients to produce what it needs. By consuming chia, you provide your brain with the all-important omega-3 ALA that it needs to function well.

✔ **Protein:** When you consume protein, it's broken down into its amino acids, which are then rebuilt into the different types of protein the brain needs to function. Chia is a complete protein — it has all nine essential amino acids that we need from our diet. These essential amino acids support the brain and can prevent decline in mood and cognitive performance. For more on protein, turn to Chapter 2.

✔ **Carbohydrates:** Carbohydrates are important for fueling the brain. When your body digests carbohydrates, they're mostly broken down into glucose, which is a simple form of sugar that provides energy. Glucose is the brain's primary energy source, but the brain can't store glucose, so it needs a steady supply of it through the bloodstream. The carbohydrates found in chia seeds release their energy slowly, allowing the brain to get the energy it needs to function well.

✔ **Antioxidants:** The brain relies on antioxidants to protect it from damage and impaired function. Oxygen balance is vital to brain health. But certain forms of oxygen, called *free radicals,* can damage brain cells through a process known as *oxidation.* Antioxidants neutralize these free radicals before they can cause any damage. Chia is high in natural antioxidants that help protect against free radicals. Vitamins, as well as the minerals iron, copper, magnesium, manganese, and zinc, are all necessary for different brain functions and are all contained in chia seeds.

Chia contains all four of these nutrients needed for brain function. Eating plenty of chia can go a long way toward supporting the nutritional requirements of your brain in conjunction with a good balanced diet.

In the following sections, we cover some of the most common brain diseases that you may be able to ward off with the nutrients found in chia.

Fighting Alzheimer's disease

Alzheimer's disease is a type of dementia that causes problems with memory, thought processes, and sometimes behavior. The symptoms are slow to develop and progressive — over time, they get worse, causing many problems with day-to-day tasks. Certain risk factors are unavoidable — such as age and family history — but diet and lifestyle are proving to be contributing factors, too, and you have control over what you eat and how you live.

Alzheimer's is caused by the death of brain cells, but what causes the death of those brain cells is still being researched. Potential risk factors include diabetes, high cholesterol, and high blood pressure. These conditions also increase the risk of stroke, which can, in turn, lead to another type of dementia.

Feeding your brain the nutrients it requires can help the brain remain strong and help you as you age. Chia has many of these nutrients that keep the brain strong, so by adding chia to your diet, you may be able to stave off Alzheimer's for a while.

Combatting depression

One in five people experience depression at some point in their lives. People suffering from depression may struggle to function on a daily basis. Sometimes they feel sad, anxious, empty, hopeless, or worried, and they often lose interest in activities they once enjoyed.

After a person is diagnosed with depression, both medication and therapy can help control it. Although it's no substitute for medication or therapy, diet can play a key role, giving the body the strength it needs to tackle deeper emotional problems.

Omega-3 fatty acids, found in chia, are needed to keep the brain healthy. People with depression appear to have lower levels of omega-3s, so consuming more omega-3s can support this deficiency.

The B vitamins are also important for nervous system function and the production of energy from food. The B vitamins are considered "anti-stress" nutrients, helping to relieve anxiety and treat depression. Niacin (vitamin B3), pyridoxine (vitamin B6), and folic acid (vitamin B9) all work with the amino acid tryptophan to produce serotonin, the "feel-good" chemical. Chia can help combat depression by supplying the nutrients your body needs to function well.

If you're suffering from depression, don't try to "self-medicate" with diet alone. Get professional help from your doctor or a licensed mental health professional.

Improving concentration

As you get tired, concentration wanes because your body doesn't have the fuel it needs to support concentration. Your mind needs energy to keep it focused. It gets energy through carbohydrates that produce glucose. Chia is a great source of carbohydrates, and it can be used as a snack at any time to help with concentration.

The carbohydrates that provide the best concentration are complex carbohydrates, not those derived from sugars. They release glucose to the body slowly, keeping you focused longer. Complex carbohydrates are the type found in chia.

The Body: Giving Your Body the Nutrients It Craves

Just like your mind has particular nutritional needs, so does your body. Individual parts of your body need to be fed specific nutrients to function properly. The types of nutrients that are critical for health and longevity include carbohydrates, proteins, fats, and vitamins and minerals. Chia is a great source of these high-quality nutrients needed for health.

In this section, we look at how feeding your body with the right nutrients can fight against common diseases. Your body needs the right foods to provide energy, to repair and support tissue growth, and to regulate metabolism.

Keeping the heart healthy

The heart pumps blood to all the tissues in the body through blood vessels and arteries. You need to keep the heart muscle, blood vessels, and arteries in good shape because the buildup of fat in these components can lead to heart disease, which can diminish quality of life or even be fatal.

Omega-3 fatty acids are key to keeping your heart healthy. Chia is the among the best plant sources of omega-3s, and it gives the heart and blood network a boost of the nutrients it needs to stay healthy.

There are other ways to keep your heart healthy, including exercise. Also, maintaining a healthy weight means the heart doesn't have to work too hard to push the blood around the body. To maintain a healthy weight, you need to be feeding your body the right nutrients, and chia can help by providing these.

In the following sections, we look at two ways you can keep your heart healthy: by lowering cholesterol and by reducing blood pressure.

Lowering cholesterol

Your body needs cholesterol to help the function of the liver. Cholesterol is a waxy, fatlike substance that is found in the cells of the body. There are two types of cholesterol that your body can produce: so-called "good" cholesterol (high-density lipoprotein, or HDL) and "bad" cholesterol (low-density lipoprotein, or LDL).

When too many fat cells build up with excess fat and other substances and cause plaque to form in your arteries, that can lead to heart disease. Most people who are diagnosed with high cholesterol can do something about it by changing their diet and lifestyle. By exercising more and eating foods high in omega-3 fatty acids, most people can lower their cholesterol levels naturally.

In every 15 g serving of chia seeds, there is an average of 3,000 mg of omega-3 ALA. Getting just one serving of chia in your daily diet goes a long way toward helping to reduce your cholesterol naturally.

Reducing blood pressure

High blood pressure is often a result of your blood vessels finding it hard to pump blood around the body because there is too much plaque build-up in the arteries. High blood pressure can lead to stroke and heart attack so it's very important to try to keep your blood pressure at a normal level. There are few symptoms of high blood pressure, but your doctor can measure your blood pressure quickly.

Like cholesterol, a healthy lifestyle and a good nutrient-dense diet can help to lower blood pressure by reducing the amount of plaque building up in your arteries. A diet high in omega-3 fatty acids, complex carbs, fiber, vitamins, and minerals can do this — and chia can help provide these nutrients. You can also help to reduce your blood pressure by lowering the intake of salt in your diet and exercising more.

Managing weight

Being overweight has a serious effect on the function of the body. Weight issues have been linked to increased risk of heart-related diseases, type-2 diabetes, cancer, and many other chronic diseases. In western society, more than 60 percent of people are overweight. Weight problems are often a result of lifestyle choices, such as consuming high-sugar drinks, processed foods, and too many calories, and not getting enough exercise.

Your body is like a car — it only needs so much fuel, and the right kind of fuel. When you overfeed your body or don't feed it the right kinds of foods, your body accumulates excess fat. The good news is, you can lose weight and help your body to support itself by changing your diet and lifestyle.

Not only are the nutrients in chia important for supporting the body, but chia also has another great benefit to support weight management. It can hold up to ten times its weight in water, meaning that when added to food, chia thickens, absorbs moisture, and hence, keeps you feeling fuller longer, so you're less likely to eat the wrong foods. Chia is also full of fiber and releases energy slowly. All these factors help in the quest to lose weight.

Helping with digestion

The digestive system is where food is broken down and distributed throughout the body for different functions. Chia holds onto water, and upon entering the stomach, it also absorbs excess stomach acid and can relieve symptoms of heartburn or indigestion.

Constipation and irritable bowel syndrome (IBS) are common digestive disorders. Chia is high in both soluble and insoluble fiber, providing a total of 5 g of fiber in every serving. This fiber helps speed up the excretion of waste and toxins from the body, preventing buildup in the intestine that could lead to disease. Many people who suffer from IBS find that chia eases symptoms immediately and helps maintain good digestive health.

Boosting energy and endurance

When the Aztecs went on marches, they brought pouches of chia that they used to sustain themselves. The Tarahumara tribe, known for their long-distance running, used chia to support themselves on their epic runs.

There are several ways in which chia helps both energy and endurance:

- ✔ **Chia is packed with complex carbs that the body needs for energy.** A 15 g serving of chia has 3 g of complex carbs, which gives you energy. The complex carbs are slow-release, which helps on the endurance side.

- ✔ **Because chia is hydrophilic, it creates a gel in the stomach and slowly releases water into the body, helping prolong hydration during endurance events.** The main problem with long-distance running or other endurance events is people's lack of ability to rehydrate, and chia is fantastic for this because it keeps the body hydrated over time.

Fighting inflammation

The average western diet gets way more omega-6 fatty acids than omega-3 fatty acids, and this high ratio of omega-6s to omega-3s has led to many inflammation-related diseases. By bringing this ratio back to 1:1, we can prevent these inflammation-based diseases. Chia has an average of 3,000 mg of omega-3s per 15 g serving, so it can go a long way toward reducing inflammation.

Other types of inflammation that can happen through exercise, wear and tear on the body, or injury to muscles and ligaments can cause inflammation of a particular area of the body. Many doctors prescribe an anti-inflammatory to get the inflammation down. Chia's unique makeup means it can act as a natural anti-inflammatory in the body.

Balancing blood sugar

Blood sugar is the amount of sugar or glucose in the blood at any given time. Balancing blood sugar is very important for optimal health, even if you don't have diabetes. A steady supply of glucose is essential for the body.

Chia can regulate the release of glucose into the system. When you eat chia, it forms a barrier inside the stomach because it forms a physical gel. This barrier helps to slow the release of glucose into the bloodstream. This is great for avoiding energy peaks and troughs that are common when eating high-sugar/low-nutrient foods (like candy bars), and it's especially helpful for diabetics, helping them control their blood sugar levels naturally.

Diabetes: Combating the fastest-growing modern lifestyle disease

There are two types of diabetes, type 1 and type 2. Type-2 diabetes is the fastest growing disease in modern society. It occurs slowly and over time. However, type-2 diabetes can be reversed if caught in time with exercise and diet. If you develop full-blown diabetes, you may require medicine or insulin for treatment.

When you have diabetes, your body doesn't have enough insulin. Insulin is a hormone of vital importance made in your pancreas. It acts like a key to open the door into your cells, letting glucose in. In diabetes, the pancreas makes too little insulin to enable all the glucose to get into the cells to produce energy. If glucose can't get into the cells, it builds up in the bloodstream. So you end up with high blood sugar levels.

Because chia seeds slow the conversion of carbohydrates into glucose, they can help people with diabetes control their blood sugar levels.

Chapter 4

The Endless Versatility of Chia

The versatility of chia is amazing. There are limitless ways to use chia in so many recipes, from your breakfast in the morning to your desserts at the end of the day, and every other meal in between. The versatility of chia in cooking helps improve the nutrient profile of the foods we eat and can be added to meals in so many different ways. Chia is easy to use as an ingredient in a variety of recipes for three key reasons:

✔ **It has a soft shell.** The soft shell means you don't have to grind it to get the nutrient value into the recipes — your body is able to absorb the valuable nutrients of chia inside the shell, without being ground down.

✔ **It's loaded with antioxidants.** The antioxidants protect the seed while it's being cooked or baked and ensure that the delicate omega-3 oils don't *oxidize* (meaning that the omega-3s don't get exposed to oxygen, causing the nutrients to diminish).

✔ **It's hydrophilic.** Chia seeds absorb up to ten times their weight in water. This means that they bulk up food (leaving you feeling full without having to consume many calories) and can act as a replacement for other less-healthy ingredients, You can do this by allowing the seeds to absorb some water to form a gel and then replace foods such as butter or eggs with chia gel, helping to improve the overall nutrient profile of any recipe.

Chia seeds are naturally gluten-free, have no known allergens, and are suitable for people on vegetarian or vegan diets, so even if you can't have a lot of other foods, you can always have chia.

In this chapter, we explain how and why chia is so versatile and can be used in almost any dish. We give you ways to cut calories, replace fat, and generally make the foods you eat a whole lot healthier. We also show you that no matter what restricted diet you're on, chia is your friend.

Enhancing Nutrients with Chia

Because chia seeds are very mild tasting and odorless, you can easily add them to all your favorite foods without affecting the flavor. So, if you're having a nutrient-poor meal, such as pasta, you can add chia to boost the nutrient profile. Instead of giving your body empty carbohydrates from the white pasta, with chia, you're adding omega-3s, fiber, protein, and antioxidants — all while enjoying the pasta you love!

There are many ways to enhance the nutrient profile of your meals with chia seeds, and that's what this section is all about.

Adding chia to everyday foods

There is no better way to improve your family's nutrition than by using chia seeds in the foods they eat every day.

Buy a shaker or just a pretty jar, fill it with chia seeds, and put it in the middle of your kitchen table. Then encourage everyone in your house to sprinkle or scoop some chia onto whatever they're eating.

Chia takes no preparation whatsoever — in fact, it's best when eaten in its raw form. Although the list of what you can add chia to is endless, here are some everyday ideas to get you started:

- Mix it into breakfast cereal.
- Spread peanut butter onto a piece of toast, and sprinkle chia seeds on top.
- Stir chia seeds into juice.
- Stir chia into yogurt.
- Toss chia over a salad.
- Sprinkle chia into soup.
- Blend chia into a smoothie.
- Bake chia into bread.
- Hide chia in a sandwich.

You won't even taste the chia seeds, but you'll know that you're getting the nutrients your body needs.

Using chia as an ingredient

Big brands are figuring out that if they add chia to foodstuffs, they can increase the nutrient profile of foods without affecting the flavor. Demand for nutritious food is growing as more people become educated about food and its effect on the body. The big brands are listening and supplying consumers with what they want. Simply by using chia as an ingredient in their branded foods, they can keep the customers who are demanding healthier options, without sacrificing any of the great taste and flavor that their customers know and love. The number of chia-spiked branded foods in the United States has risen greatly in recent years. Today, you can find chia bread, chia pizzas, chia cookies, chia chips — you name it!

It's not just the big companies that can add chia to their recipes. At home, you can easily add chia to all your favorite recipes. Next time you're making grandma's bread recipe, throw in a few scoops of whole or milled chia seeds. No one will notice the difference in taste, but they'll be getting plenty of valuable nutrients to keep them healthy on the inside.

Including chia in your favorite drinks

One of the oldest chia recipes — it's been around for centuries — is chia fresca. This drink is common in Mexico and Central America. You simply add chia to water, lemon juice, and sugar. The Mexican cultures knew that chia seeds were great for energy and used chia fresca as a refreshing drink to refuel their bodies.

Drinking chia is a great way to get the valuable nutrients into your system fast. Throw a couple spoonfuls of chia into your morning juice or add them to your blended smoothies (see Chapter 8) to get some great nutrition into your favorite drinks. You could even try them in a cocktail!

If you're an athlete, adding chia to your water helps to rehydrate you by slowly releasing the water through the gel that the chia water forms in your stomach. This can help you exercise for longer because it prolongs hydration needed for endurance sports.

When chia is added to water, the chia absorbs the water and creates a gel. If you put too much chia in a drink, it may get too thick. Play around to get the consistency that works best for you.

Using chia gel

Chia gel (chia and fluid) can be used in several ways and has several benefits. Probably the best benefit is that it slows the conversion of carbohydrates into sugars, thereby regulating healthy blood sugar levels, which in turn helps with energy levels.

A good rule of thumb for creating a gel is six parts water to one part seeds. Simply pour the water into a bowl, mix well, and let it sit for a few minutes. Then mix again and let it stand for ten minutes, mix again, and use as necessary. Chia gel can be added to all your favorite foods.

You can make chia gel using any liquid you choose — you're not limited to just water. Good liquids to try are coconut milk (which makes a deliciously creamy gel and is fantastic added to curries or used as a base for puddings), coconut water (great if you want a real health kick with added electrolytes), or any other milk, nut milk, or non-dairy substitute.

Using Chia as a Substitute

In the preceding section, we talk about enhancing your recipes by adding chia to them. But you can also take out ingredients, and replace them with chia. This can greatly improve the recipe's nutrient value — because typically you're taking out not-so-healthy foods and replacing them with the super-nutritious chia.

For example, common recipes that are traditionally baked using butter and eggs can be made healthier by reducing the amount of butter and eggs and using chia gel instead. Thanks to its gelling capabilities, chia can be used in the baking process as a binding agent instead of eggs or as a fat replacement.

In this section, we tell you all about how to use chia to replace common ingredients in your favorite recipes.

Using chia instead of eggs

If you want to cut down on eggs, you have an egg allergy, or you're following a vegan diet, you can use chia seeds instead of eggs in most recipes.

You need milled chia seeds, so either buy them milled from a shop or grind the seeds yourself using a coffee grinder. Then just mix 1 tablespoon milled chia seeds with 3 tablespoons water to replace one egg. Do this for each egg that the recipe calls for.

Eggs are used so often in baking for a few reasons:

✔ To bind the ingredients and make them all stick together.

✔ To add moisture to the baked goods and help to keep them from drying out.

✔ To help the baked goods rise. When you beat the eggs, air is added, and in the baking process the air heats and expands, making the baked item rise.

Chia acts as an egg on all three fronts, thanks to its gelling capabilities and oil content.

Using chia instead of butter

Most of the fats called for in recipes (for example, butter) are high in saturated fat, which can be bad for your heart. You can use chia in place of some of the butter in many baking recipes.

Chia has a fat content of 30 percent, but it's the kind of fat that's good for your heart.

Bulking up your favorite recipes with chia

Bulking up your meals is the best way to stretch your calorie budget and a great way to improve the nutrition of your favorite dishes. You know when you're trying to be healthy, so you cook your favorite recipe, but eat a smaller portion, and then you end up dissatisfied and wanting more and more.

Instead of avoiding your favorite recipes, look at ways to bulk them up by adding chia, fruits, or vegetables. Not only do you get to enjoy your favorite recipes, but you feel fuller and happier. Here are some examples of how to bulk up your favorite recipes using chia:

✔ When eating pizza, put loads of vegetables and chia on it instead of meat.

✔ If you want to eat a casserole, fill it with vegetables and chia.

✔ When eating cereal, pour a little less into your bowl and add chia gel to bulk it up.

✔ Make homemade burgers, but use half the meat that the recipe calls for and use chia gel as a replacement for the missing meat.

✔ Mix chia gel into cream cheese before you spread it on your bagel.

✔ Add chia gel to your pancake mix.

✔ Use chia gel in all your baked goods.

To replace butter in a recipe, simply make a chia gel (see "Using chia gel," earlier in this chapter). Use chia gel instead of half the butter that a recipe needs. So, for instance, if a recipe calls for 1 cup butter, use ½ cup butter and ½ cup chia gel. It won't affect the taste of the recipe, but it will greatly improve the nutrient value and reduce the amount of saturated fat.

With chia, you can have your cake and eat it, too!

Seeing How Chia Plays Nice with All Kinds of Dietary Restrictions

Today, many people are on specialized diets. Maybe they've gone gluten-free, or they're vegan, or they avoid certain foods because of allergies. Whatever foods you like, don't like, have to avoid, or want to avoid, chia has you covered. Its versatility means that it can be used by almost everybody as a way to boost nutrition and improve health!

In this section we show you that no matter what foods you have to avoid in your diet, chia is probably not one of them.

Eliminating or cutting back on animal products

Many people want to avoid all animal products for ethical and/or health reasons, but they may find it hard to do because so many of the foods we eat come from animals. Even if you avoid meat, many other foods are made with animal products.

Chia is grown and harvested without the use of any animals or animal byproducts, so it can help provide some of the nutrients that traditionally come from animals in the diet. It's high in omega-3 fatty acids, so if you're avoiding fish, you can use chia as your source of omega-3s. It's also a complete protein, so nutritionally, it's great for people who don't eat meat.

If you're trying to reduce or eliminate animal products from your diet, using chia can give you some of the nutrients you need.

 For more information, check out *Living Vegan For Dummies* and *Vegan Cooking For Dummies,* both by Alexandra Jamieson (Wiley). And for a vegetarian diet, check out *Living Vegetarian For Dummies,* 2nd Edition, and *Vegetarian Cooking For Dummies,* both by Suzanne Havala Hobbs (Wiley).

Gluten, gluten, gone!

Unless you've been living under a rock, you're probably aware of the gluten-free foods sweeping the nation. Every time you turn around, somebody's talking about eliminating gluten from her diet. Gluten is a protein found in wheat. People who suffer from celiac disease have no tolerance for gluten and have to follow a very strict gluten-free diet. The disease affects the digestive system, and sufferers can get chronic diarrhea, bloating, excess gas, and upset stomachs if they ingest even the tiniest amount of gluten. Plenty of people who *don't* suffer from celiac disease are also going gluten-free because they believe it's healthier.

Whether you choose not to include gluten in your diet by choice or because you need to avoid gluten at all costs, chia can be a valued addition to your diet. Chia is naturally gluten-free and is highly nutritious, so when you're trying to figure out how to alter your diet to support going gluten-free, chia can serve as a foundation for many recipes.

In Chapter 11, we cover special diets and offer a few gluten-free recipes. For much more information on going gluten-free, check out *Living Gluten-Free For Dummies,* 2nd Edition, by Danna Korn (Wiley). And for more recipes, try *Gluten-Free Cooking For Dummies,* 2nd Edition, by Danna Korn, and *Gluten-Free Baking For Dummies,* by Dr. Jean McFadden Layton and Linda Larsen (both published by Wiley).

Combating allergies

There are so many foods that people are allergic to today, and the list seems to be getting longer and longer. Maybe it's the increased use of genetically modified foods throughout the world, or maybe we're being so cautious about everything these days that we develop more allergic reactions, but whatever the reason, people need to avoid more and more foods all the time.

Nuts are common foods that people are allergic to, as is gluten (see the preceding section), and of course many people need to avoid dairy. The list goes on. . . .

Thankfully, chia seeds are nowhere near that list because it has no known allergens. Many humans have never shown an allergic reaction to chia because we've been eating chia since ancient times. In any case, nearly everyone can benefit from the goodness of chia and all the nutrients and health benefits that the tiny seeds provide. So, go ahead and add chia to your diet and make sure to check out the recipes in this book to get inspiration for what to do with your chia seeds!

Chapter 5

Buying, Storing, and Using Chia

*W*hen you're getting ready to cook with chia, you need to start with the basics: good-quality seeds. In this chapter, we tell you what to look for. We also walk you through the various types of chia you may find on your grocery store shelves. Then we tell you how to store chia in your kitchen, and how to prepare it for consumption. Finally, we fill you in on how to stock your kitchen so that you're ready to cook!

This chapter lays the groundwork for all kinds of delicious and nutritious chia meals.

Shopping for Chia Seeds

All chia is not created equal. Chia seeds require very specific growing conditions for the seeds to become high in omega-3 fatty acids, protein, and other nutrients. Weather conditions, the amount of sunlight, and temperature are just a few of the factors at play to ensure that the seeds harvested are highly nutritious.

Then there are the harvesting and cleaning techniques used. These techniques differ immensely from one chia producer to another, and they contribute to the quality of the resulting chia seeds.

The difference in appearance between good-quality chia and inferior chia is very slight, unless you know what you're looking for. Because of the difference in nutritional value between good chia and inferior chia, it pays to know what to look for when you shop.

The chia cleaning process

All chia has to go through a cleaning process before it can show up on your grocery store shelves. The cleaning process never involves chemicals — just a series of mechanical systems.

Chia is harvested different ways — sometimes by hand and sometimes by heavy-duty machinery — but no matter how it's harvested, weed seeds and plant parts need to be removed. This is done is by using sieves or screens.

Other seeds such as amaranth grow alongside chia, and they're often harvested with chia. Amaranth is a weed and although it does have other essential nutrients, it's not chia and shouldn't be sold as chia. To remove the amaranth seeds from chia, finer screens are used to separate out these seeds. Amaranth seeds are smaller than chia, black in color, and completely round, so if the chia you buy contains a lot of these weed seeds, shop around for another brand.

High-quality chia seeds are approximately 2 mm long and are either black or white in color. They can be a dark gray color or a creamy white color, but they're never brown.

If you see chia that has lots of brown seeds in it, don't buy it. Brown seeds are immature — they don't have the high levels of omega-3 fatty acids, protein, or antioxidants expected from chia.

In general, good-quality chia contains mostly black seeds with a few white seeds speckled amongst them. However, there are all white seeds available, which are high quality and just as nutritious as the black ones. As long as the chia you buy has no brown or very few brown seeds, you can be sure that you're buying fully mature seeds that are full of the nutrients you expect.

Recognizing the Various Types of Chia

Chia always comes from the plant, *Salvia hispanica* L, but by the time it makes it to your grocery store shelves, it can be presented in different forms.

In this section, we tell you about ground or milled chia, white chia, and chia that has been hydrated prior to sale.

Ground or milled chia

Whole chia seeds are what come naturally form the *Salvia hispanica* L plant. These tiny black and white seeds can be eaten whole. However, chia is sometimes sold as milled or ground seed. When chia is milled, it's done using very specialized milling machinery that doesn't get hot during the milling process. This is to ensure that the omega-3 oils aren't damaged in any way.

Organic or not?

You may see organic chia at your local market, but is the non-organic "worse"? The chia plant is a member of the mint family, so insects are naturally reluctant to come near it. That means that crops of chia are never sprayed with pesticides. Most of the chia available is naturally grown, without chemicals, but it isn't certified organic because of the costs involved in that certification process.

Getting the certificates and ensuring that the fields used to grow chia were never used before for sprayed crops is very expensive and increases the price of chia greatly. Even

then, the organic chia available, although it's organic, can be of inferior quality with low levels of nutrients.

To complicate things further, some chia is labeled "organic" or "organically grown" when it isn't. The black market for organic certificates is rife, and companies can just use these terms for marketing purposes.

Instead of focusing on the label *organic,* look for high-quality chia that's black or white in color. You'll come out ahead.

The only reason chia is sold in milled form is to satisfy people's preference for texture. Milled chia can also be used instead of or mixed with other flours. Whole and milled chia seeds are the exact same nutritionally, but some people simply prefer a powder-like texture because it can be stirred into liquid or foods and it completely disappears. Milled chia seeds are great in smoothies or for sneaking chia into kids' food.

It really doesn't matter which you choose to use — milled or whole seeds. Both are highly nutritious and easily absorbable.

The only disadvantage with buying ground or milled chia is that you can't see the quality of the seeds. You can't tell if the milled seed was made up of immature brown seeds before it was milled. For this reason, it pays to buy your chia seeds from a reputable brand such as Chia bia or AZChia.

You can grind your own seeds at home using a coffee grinder. This way, you can ensure that your milled chia is coming from high-quality seeds.

White chia

Some brands of chia sell only white chia seeds. They're able to do this by isolating the few white seeds that occur naturally throughout the black. They then plant only these seeds, which produce crops having only white chia seeds.

The white seeds are comparable to the black nutritionally. The black seeds are a tiny bit higher in antioxidants.

Some people like the white seeds because the color isn't as pronounced in foods — white disappears more easily than black. Usually, the white seeds are more expensive than the black, so if you're buying chia and you don't care about the color, you might as well choose the black seeds.

Pre-hydrated chia

You may see pre-hydrated chia seeds on the market. This just means that the seeds have already absorbed liquid. You're more likely to see this in drinks, puddings, and other foods that are already mixed with chia and ready to use.

Chia has been a great addition to sports drinks. Many different chia-enhanced drinks are on the market, helping athletes prolong hydration, increase endurance, and speed muscle recovery. For athletes who prefer less sugar and want to avoid synthetic ingredients, these chia sports drinks are beneficial. Just be sure to look at the other ingredients in the drinks to ensure that you're not getting not too much sugar or additives alongside the chia.

Pre-hydrated chia seeds don't last as long as the dry seeds, so pay attention to the use-by dates.

Storing Chia Seeds

After the seeds are harvested, chia can be stored for up to five years while retaining its nutrients. Store your chia seeds in a sealed bag at room temperature, away from direct sunlight. Glass containers are also ideal for storing chia seeds.

You don't need to refrigerate chia seeds — their naturally occurring antioxidants help chia seeds retain all the nutrients.

Preparing Chia to Eat

The real beauty about chia is its ease of use. It's never been easier to fill your belly with omega-3s, protein, fiber, and antioxidants. All you need is a bag of chia! You can do any or all of the following with chia seeds:

✔ **Shake it** over cereals, salads, stir-fries, chopped fruit, granola, peanut butter, jams, and spreads.

> - **Stir it** through yogurts, puddings, custards, casseroles, curries, salad dressings, oatmeal, stews, and lentils.
> - **Blend it** into smoothies, baby purees, soups, juice drinks, and pasta sauces.
> - **Bake it** into cakes, brownies, cookies, granola bars, muffins, pancakes, waffles, and bread.

You can cook with chia up to 350 degrees. This means that you can use it in most of your favorite baked goods recipes. It can also be used as a substitute for eggs and butter, which allows you to reduce the fat and calories to make healthier breads, cakes, and other goodies. We discuss how to do this in Chapter 4 and give you some great baking recipes in Part IV.

You can also make chia gel that you can use in all kinds of recipes. Turn to Chapter 4 for instructions on making chia gel.

Stocking Your Kitchen

When your kitchen is well stocked with all the tools and ingredients you need, cooking is a lot easier. You're more likely to cook a healthy meal when you don't have to go to the grocery store for something basic.

Get rid of the clutter in your kitchen and have the essentials on hand, close to where you cook. This way, you won't spend precious cooking time looking for that pot in the back of the cupboard that you have to move a dozen things to get to.

In this section, we give you a basic list of kitchen essentials — from pots and pans, to knives and chopping boards. We also tell you what ingredients to have on hand to make cooking a breeze.

Equipment

When it comes to decking out your kitchen with essential equipment, it pays to invest as much as you can afford on good-quality stainless-steel pots and pans. These tools will not only prevent your food from sticking but also help you keep your cool in the kitchen. Knives are another important investment — a few good-quality knives will make chopping and carving much easier.

If you have to choose what to invest in, knives and pots are where you should spend your money.

The following list covers the basics you need to make sure you're well-prepared for all the recipes in this book and more:

- ✔ Pots and pans
  - Three saucepans with lids — one large, one medium, and one small
  - Large frying pan
  - Wok
  - Large Dutch oven or ovenproof casserole with lid
  - Griddle
  - Two large nonstick baking sheets
  - Large high-sided roasting pan
- ✔ Knives
  - Large chef's knife
  - Small paring knife
  - Bread knife
- ✔ Electric tools
  - Food processor
  - Blender
  - Hand blender
  - Electric kettle
- ✔ Utensils
  - Three different wooden spoons
  - Slotted spoon
  - Three large serving spoons
  - Fish turner
  - Spatula
  - Whisk
  - Potato masher
  - Ladle
  - Grater (coarse and fine)
  - Pastry brush
  - Speed peeler

> - Garlic crusher
> - Tongs
> - Kitchen scissors
> - Rolling pin
> - Sieve

✔ Other

> - Assortment of mixing bowls
> - Colander/steamer
> - 9-x-13-inch baking dish
> - Angel food cake pan
> - Spring-form tin
> - Muffin pans
> - Chopping boards (one for meat, one for vegetables)

✔ Measuring tools

> - Set of measuring cups (1 cup, ½ cup, ⅓ cup, ¼ cup)
> - Set of measuring spoons (1 tablespoon, 1 teaspoon, ½ teaspoon, ¼ teaspoon)
> - Large glass measuring cup
> - Kitchen scale

Ingredients

A well-stocked pantry gets you well on the way to cooking nutritious meals without too much heartache. If you have the essentials on hand, you're always ready to whip up something delicious and nutritious without having to think.

This section is all about what you should stock up on to make your food taste great.

Nonperishable foodstuff

There are so many different types of grains, legumes, and flours that are nonperishable — you can stock up on these dry goods and be ready to cook any time. There are also some great canned fish and vegetables that can add value to your meals.

We recommend you always have the following in your cupboard:

- **Rice:** Arborio rice, basmati rice, brown rice
- **Pasta:** Fusilli, lasagna, linguine, macaroni, penne, spaghetti
- **Grains:** Bulgur, couscous, oatmeal, pearl barley
- **Legumes:** Butter beans, cannelloni beans, chickpeas, kidney beans, lentils (red and green)
- **Seeds:** Chia seeds (whole and milled), pumpkin seeds, sunflower seeds
- **Nuts:** Almonds, cashews, hazelnuts, pecans, pine nuts
- **Baking essentials:** All-purpose flour, baking powder, brown sugar (soft), cocoa powder, confectioner's sugar, cornstarch, super-fine sugar, whole-wheat flour, yeast (dried)
- **Canned goods:** Anchovies, olives, sweet corn, tomatoes (chopped), tuna
- **Other:** Apricots (dried), coconut milk, honey, pure maple syrup, raisins (regular and golden), stock cubes (beef, chicken, and vegetable), vinegar (balsamic, red wine, and white wine)

Herbs and spices

To bring flavor to your meals, you need to add spices or herbs or a mixture of both. By using herbs and spices, you can cut down on the amount of salt that you use in cooking. Some recipes in this book call for fresh herbs, but buying just a small bunch of herbs can be expensive, so it's often easier to use dried herbs. The basic rule is that 1 teaspoon of dried herbs is equal to 1 tablespoon of fresh, more or less.

If you like the idea of using fresh herbs, you can grow the basics — such as parsley, rosemary, and thyme — on your kitchen windowsill.

Here's our basic list of the herbs and spices you should have on hand:

- Allspice
- Basil (dried)
- Bay leaves
- Chili (flakes and powder)
- Cilantro (seeds and ground)
- Cloves (whole)
- Cumin (seeds and ground)
- Curry powder
- Cinnamon (ground)
- Fennel (seeds)

- Ginger (ground)
- Marjoram (dried)
- Mustard (seeds and powder)
- Oregano (dried)
- Paprika (smoked)
- Parsley (dried)
- Pepper, black (whole peppercorns)
- Pepper, white (ground)
- Rosemary (dried)
- Sage (dried)
- Sea salt
- Thyme (dried)
- Turmeric

Dried herbs and spices lose their potency and shouldn't be used for more than a year, so keep an eye on your supply and toss them after a year.

Sauces and condiments

Sauces make meals wonderful, and chia is a fantastic addition to any sauce — especially milled chia, because you can mix it into sauces, add a little water, and the flavor of the sauce stays the same.

We recommend you always have the following sauces on hand:

- Curry paste (red and green)
- Fish sauce
- Ketchup
- Mustard (English)
- Oyster sauce
- Soy sauce
- Tabasco sauce
- Teriyaki sauce
- Worcestershire sauce

Oils and spreads

Oils and spreads are where people often go wrong. If you use too much butter or cheap oils, you increase your risk of developing heart disease. The good news is, the kinds of healthy oils available is increasing all the time.

If you do use oils and spreads, choose healthier versions and try to cut down on the amount you use. Try using cooking spray instead of oil when frying. Use olive oil on bread instead of butter. Coconut oil is great for cooking because it's stable at high temperatures and free from trans fats; it can also be used as a tasty spread instead of butter. Rapeseed oil is good for cooking as well as in dressings.

Avoid any spread that has a long list of ingredients that you don't recognize.

We recommend having the following oils and spreads in your pantry:

- ✔ Coconut oil
- ✔ Olive oil (extra virgin and regular)
- ✔ Peanut oil
- ✔ Pesto (red and green)
- ✔ Rapeseed oil
- ✔ Sesame oil
- ✔ Tapenade

Frozen foods

Some fruits and vegetables are just as good, if not better, when they're frozen. This is because they're picked at exactly the right time, when they're naturally ripe. They're frozen immediately, helping to retain the nutrients.

The freezer is also handy for keeping pastry so you don't have to make it fresh every time. Make a batch of pastry, replacing some of the flour with milled chia seeds, and then freeze it to use whenever you like.

We also recommend freezing extra soups or stews that you've made using chia seeds so you have them on hand for a fast, nutritious meal.

The following foods are handy to keep in your freezer:

- ✔ Bananas
- ✔ Phyllo pastry
- ✔ Peas
- ✔ Puff pastry
- ✔ Raspberries
- ✔ Strawberries
- ✔ Sweet corn

Part II

Starting Your Day the Right Way: Breakfasts

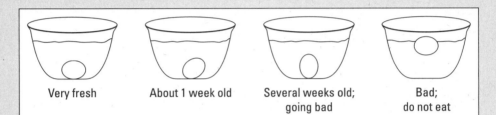

Very fresh   About 1 week old   Several weeks old;   Bad;
                                  going bad   do not eat

© John Wiley & Sons, Inc.

Find out more about making chia puddings in an article at www.dummies.com/extras/cookingwithchia.

In this part . . .

✔ Prepare great-tasting breakfast bowls that are full of nutrients and easy to make, and that help keep you feeling full until lunchtime.

✔ Uncover the power of mixing oats with chia seeds.

✔ Discover delicious weekend recipes for when you have a little more time in the mornings.

✔ Find the best ways of getting as many nutrients as possible into smoothie recipes, along with alternatives for dairy and sugar.

Chapter 6

Getting Chia into Your Breakfast Bowl

You've heard it before: Breakfast is the most important meal of the day. But it's also the meal that's most often skipped. Mornings are usually hectic, especially if there are kids in the house who need to eat and get out the door to school. The easiest and quickest solution is often to throw something into a bowl and get on with your day. However, many of the breakfast cereals on your grocery store's shelves are full of sugar and aren't the healthiest choices.

This chapter is all about preparing breakfast bowls that are not only nutritious and delicious but also easy to prepare and quick to grab on busy mornings. Using chia to add extra nutrients to your breakfast bowls is a fantastic way to set you up for the day. The seeds are slow to convert from carbohydrates to sugars, so they provide you with sustained energy throughout the day and keep you feeling full until lunch.

Chia and Oats: A Powerful Breakfast

When it comes to packing in the nutrients at breakfast time, you can't get much better than mixing chia seeds with oats. The combined nutrients in chia and oats will get you well on your way to filling up on the daily nutrients needed to give you sustained energy, keep your heart healthy, and keep your digestive system running smoothly. The recipes in this section are all highly nutritious, and some can be made in advance, so you can easily grab a quick breakfast bowl of oats and chia as you run out the door!

Banana and Cinnamon Porridge

Prep time: 10 min • **Cook time:** 25 min • **Yield:** 4 servings

Ingredients	Directions
4 cups 2 percent milk	*1* In a medium saucepan, bring the milk to a boil.
1 cup steel-cut Irish oatmeal	
½ teaspoon salt	*2* Sprinkle in the oatmeal, stirring constantly to prevent any lumps from forming.
¼ cup whole chia seeds	
2 ripe bananas, finely sliced	*3* Add the salt, and turn down the heat.
½ teaspoon ground cinnamon	*4* Simmer for 25 minutes, stirring occasionally to give you a smooth creamy porridge.
2 tablespoons desiccated coconut	
4 tablespoons pure maple syrup	*5* Take the porridge off the heat, and stir the chia seeds evenly throughout the mixture.
	6 Divide evenly between 4 serving bowls, and top with the banana.
	7 Sprinkle cinnamon and coconut over each serving.
	8 Drizzle maple syrup over each serving.

Per serving: Calories 443 (From Fat 111); Fat 12g (Saturated 6g); Cholesterol 20mg; Sodium 415mg; Carbohydrate 71g (Dietary Fiber 9g); Protein 34g.

Note: You can keep any leftover porridge covered in the fridge for another day. Simply add some milk or water and heat in the microwave until warm.

Overnight Oats

Prep time: 10 min • **Yield:** 1 serving

Ingredients	Directions
½ cup old-fashioned oatmeal	*1* In a medium bowl, combine the oatmeal, chia, yogurt, almond milk, and stevia; mix well.
1 tablespoon whole chia seeds	
½ cup plain nonfat Greek yogurt	*2* Spoon half the mixture into a 12-ounce glass jar.
½ cup unsweetened vanilla almond milk	*3* Add 1 tablespoon of raspberries to the jar. Then add the remaining oat mixture to the jar, and top it off with the remaining raspberries.
Stevia, to taste	
3 tablespoons fresh raspberries	*4* Seal the jar and allow it to sit in the refrigerator overnight.
	5 In the morning, grab the jar for a nutritious breakfast.

Per serving: Calories 313 (From Fat 68); Fat 8g (Saturated 1g); Cholesterol 0mg; Sodium 126mg; Carbohydrate 45g (Dietary Fiber 8g); Protein 20g.

Tip: If the mixture is too thick in the morning, add some extra almond milk.

Vary It! Instead of using store-bought almond milk, you can make your own. Check out the simple recipe for almond milk in the "Nutty nut milks" sidebar, later in this chapter.

Variations on a theme

Try any of the following variations for a different taste each morning. Simply mix the ingredients together, and replace the raspberries in the Overnight Oats recipe with the following suggestions:

✔ **Peachy Peaches:** 2 small peaches, diced; ¼ teaspoon cinnamon; and a drizzle of honey

✔ **Strawberry Bliss:** 8 strawberries, sliced; and 1 tablespoon strawberry jam

✔ **Banana and Peanut:** 1 medium banana, sliced; 1 tablespoon peanut butter; and a drizzle of honey

✔ **Chocolate Cherry:** 1 tablespoon chocolate chips and 1 tablespoon dried sour cherries

✔ **Nutty Surprise:** 1 tablespoon pecan nuts, 1 tablespoon desiccated coconut, ¼ teaspoon cinnamon, and 1 tablespoon pure maple syrup

✔ **Apple and Pecan:** 1 medium apple (cored and chopped), 1 tablespoon chopped pecans, and a drizzle of honey or pure maple syrup

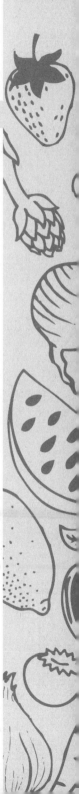

Classic Granola

Prep time: 10 min • **Cook time:** 40 min • **Yield:** 12 servings

Ingredients	Directions
5 cups oatmeal	**1** Preheat the oven to 300 degrees.
2 tablespoons cashews	
2 tablespoons almonds	**2** In a large bowl, mix the oatmeal, cashews, almonds, peanuts, pistachios, pecans, Brazil nuts, walnuts, pumpkin seeds, sunflower seeds, salt, cinnamon, ginger, and stevia.
2 tablespoons peanuts	
2 tablespoons pistachios	
2 tablespoons pecans	**3** Add the cashew butter and sunflower oil.
1 tablespoon Brazil nuts	
1 tablespoon walnuts	**4** Stir well, and spread out over 2 large baking sheets.
2 tablespoons pumpkin seeds	
2 tablespoons sunflower seeds	**5** Bake in the oven for 30 to 40 minutes, stirring at 15 minutes and again at 25 minutes.
½ teaspoon salt	**6** Stop baking when the granola begins to smell good and looks golden. It won't be crunchy at first.
½ teaspoon ground cinnamon	
½ teaspoon ground ginger	**7** Allow to cool and pour into a large bowl.
½ cup stevia	
4 tablespoons cashew butter	**8** Add the chia and raisins.
6 tablespoons sunflower oil	
½ cup whole chia seeds	**9** Store in an airtight container, and enjoy for up to 2 weeks.
½ cup raisins	

Per serving: Calories 333 (From Fat 174); Fat 20g (Saturated 3g); Cholesterol 0mg; Sodium 122mg; Carbohydrate 34g (Dietary Fiber 7g); Protein 9g.

Tip: Try eating your granola served with a dollop of plain yogurt and a drizzle of honey.

High-Fiber Bulgur Breakfast Fix

Prep time: 10 min • **Cook time:** 20 min • **Yield:** 4 servings

Ingredients	Directions
1 cup coarse bulgur wheat	**1** In a medium saucepan, bring water to a boil and add the bulgur wheat. Simmer the bulgur for 15 to 18 minutes, until tender.
1½ cups 2 percent milk	
¼ cup rolled oats	
15 dried figs, chopped	**2** Meanwhile, in a separate medium saucepan, heat the milk over medium heat and add the rolled oats. Bring the oats to a boil; then simmer gently for 5 minutes or according to the package instructions. Set aside.
¼ cup chopped pecans	
3 tablespoons pure maple syrup	
4 tablespoons whole chia seeds	**3** Drain the cooked bulgur and return it to its saucepan over low heat.
2 medium apples, cut into chunks	**4** Drain the figs into the bulgur, squeezing out any excess water in the figs using the back of a spoon.
4 tablespoons raisins	**5** Add the figs, cooked oats, pecans, maple syrup, and chia; stir well.
	6 Divide the mixture evenly between 4 serving bowls and top each serving with the apples and raisins.

Per serving: Calories 480 (From Fat 101); Fat 11g (Saturated 2g); Cholesterol 7mg; Sodium 59mg; Carbohydrate 90g (Dietary Fiber 17g); Protein 12g.

Note: You can keep any leftover bulgur wheat covered in the fridge for up to 3 days. Simply add some milk or water and heat in the microwave until warm.

The lowdown on bulgur

Bulgur is a form of whole wheat that has been cleaned, partially cooked, dried, and then ground into grains of different sizes. The resulting grain has a mild nutty flavor when cooked and is a great source of protein, iron, magnesium, and B vitamins. The main benefit of bulgur wheat is its high fiber content. One cup of cooked bulgur wheat has a massive 8 g of fiber! Bulgur's fiber content is the main reason more people are substituting bulgur for rice. Bulgur is the main ingredient in the Middle Eastern salad tabbouleh.

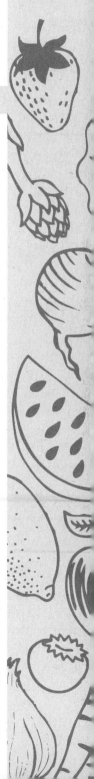

Mega Muesli

Prep time: 15 min • **Yield:** 8 servings

Ingredients	Directions
3 cups rolled oats	*1* In a large bowl, combine all the ingredients and mix well.
½ cup dried cherries	
½ cup raisins	*2* Transfer the muesli to an airtight glass container (Kilner jars work great for this purpose) and use as and when desired.
½ cup unsweetened cranberries	
½ cup dried mango, chopped	
½ cup hazelnuts	
½ cup pecans, chopped	
½ cup flaked almonds	
½ cup desiccated coconut	
½ cup pumpkin seeds	
½ cup sunflower seeds	
½ cup whole chia seeds	
¼ cup stevia	

Per serving: Calories 533 (From Fat 267); Fat 30g (Saturated 6g); Cholesterol 0mg; Sodium 21mg; Carbohydrate 59g (Dietary Fiber 11g); Protein 13g.

Tip: This muesli is great served with your favorite ice-cold milk.

Tip: To make more muesli so that the whole family can enjoy as much as they like for longer, simply double or triple the ingredients. The muesli will last months if kept in an airtight container in a cool, dark place.

A brief history of muesli

A Swiss physician by the name of Maximilian Bircher-Benner first introduced muesli to his hospital patients around 1900 as part of their therapy. He believed that a diet rich in fresh fruits and vegetables was essential. Muesli was inspired by a dish Bircher-Benner and his wife had been served while on a hike in the Swiss Alps. However, muesli didn't become popular in western societies until the 1960s, when there was an increased interest in health food and vegetarian diets. Since then, muesli has become a popular choice the world over as a quick and nutritious morning meal.

Chia Breakfast Fruit Bowl

Prep time: 15 min • **Yield:** 3 servings

Ingredients	Directions
1 medium ripe banana	**1** Peel and slice the banana, and put in a large bowl.
1 medium apple	
2 small peaches	**2** Core the apple, and chop it into small pieces; add it to the bowl with the bananas.
1 pink grapefruit	
½ cup grapes	**3** Halve the peaches, remove the stones, and thinly slice the peaches; add them to the bowl.
10 strawberries	
½ cup raspberries	**4** Peel the grapefruit and cut it into segments, removing any excess pulp that doesn't look appealing to eat; add it to the bowl.
½ cup blueberries	
½ cup orange juice	
1 cup nonfat plain Greek yogurt	**5** Wash the grapes and cut them in half; add them to the bowl.
1 cup rolled oats	**6** Wash and cut the strawberries in quarters; add them to the bowl.
2 tablespoons whole chia seeds	
Honey, to taste	**7** Wash the raspberries and blueberries; add them to the bowl.
	8 In the large bowl, mix all the fruit well.
	9 Pour the orange juice onto the fruit, and stir.
	10 Divide the fruit between 3 bowls, and add yogurt on top of each serving. Sprinkle oats and chia on top of each serving. Drizzle with honey and enjoy a delicious, nutritious breakfast bowl.

Per serving: Calories 376 (From Fat 44); Fat 5g (Saturated 1g); Cholesterol 0mg; Sodium 32mg; Carbohydrate 76g (Dietary Fiber 12g); Protein 14g.

Note: Eat this breakfast immediately after preparing it — the fruits don't keep well.

Vary It! You can use any fruits you like in this recipe, so choose fruits that are in season and look good to eat.

Healthy Breakfast Puddings and Yogurts

Whoever said that you couldn't have pudding for breakfast hadn't heard of chia pudding! When you make pudding with chia, it makes a delicious and nutritious breakfast. Chia puddings are a great way to start your day. You can prepare them in advance and grab them in the morning to bring to work, eat them en route, or have them as a midmorning snack.

Another breakfast staple is yogurt. Yogurts can be a great addition to a healthy diet by providing calcium for healthy bones, and probiotics to help keep the immune system healthy.

Nutty nut milks

People have consumed traditional animal milks (like cow's milk and goat's milk) as a source of nutrition for many years, but they're becoming less popular as more people discover they have food sensitivities and allergies. More and more, nutritionists and dietitians are recommending nut milks as alternatives to animal milks. Nut milks have many essential vitamins and minerals and not as much saturated fats as animal milks do.

You can buy a nut milk such as almond milk in your local grocery store, but you can also make your own! To make your own almond milk, you'll need the following ingredients:

- 1 cup raw almonds
- 2 cups water
- Stevia, to taste

To prepare the almond milk, follow these steps:

1. **Fill a large bowl with water, and add the almonds to the bowl; allow them to soak overnight or up to 2 days.**

2. **Drain and rinse the almonds.**

3. **In a blender, combine the almonds and water, and blend for 2 minutes.**

4. **Strain the mixture through a nut bag, squeezing the bag.**

   Note: A nut bag is a small bag made of porous material. You put a blended nut and water mixture into the nut bag, and then squeeze through the liquid to make nut milks. You can pick up a nut bag in health food stores or online.

5. **Sweeten the resulting liquid with stevia to taste.**

You can store the almond milk in an airtight container in the fridge for up to two days.

Basic Chia Pudding

Prep time: 10 min • **Yield:** 2 servings

Ingredients	Directions
1 cup coconut milk (from a carton)	*1* In a large bowl, add the coconut milk and almond milk.
1 cup unsweetened almond milk	*2* Whisk in the maple syrup until fully combined.
2 tablespoons pure maple syrup	*3* Add the chia, cinnamon, and salt, and whisk again until fully combined.
4 tablespoons whole chia seeds	
¼ teaspoon ground cinnamon	*4* Split the mixture between 2 serving bowls and cover with plastic wrap.
Pinch of salt	
	5 Allow the bowls to sit in the refrigerator for at least 4 hours, whisking occasionally. For best results, leave to sit overnight.

Per serving: Calories 207 (From Fat 90); Fat 10g (Saturated 3g); Cholesterol 0mg; Sodium 156mg; Carbohydrate 27g (Dietary Fiber 8g); Protein 4g.

Note: This pudding recipe will keep covered in the refrigerator for up to 5 days, so if you want to make a larger batch for the whole family to enjoy throughout the week, simply double or triple the ingredients.

Vary It! Instead of using store-bought almond milk, try to make your own. Check out the simple recipe for almond milk in the "Nutty nut milks" sidebar, earlier in this section.

Vary It! This is a very basic pudding recipe that can be infinitely varied. If you don't like cinnamon, try vanilla extract instead. If you don't like coconut milk or almond milk, swap them for your favorite dairy milk or other nut milk. If you like a sweeter pudding, add some stevia, honey, or any sweetener you love. The key to chia pudding is experimenting to find what you like.

Tip: Fruit is the perfect accompaniment to this basic chia pudding recipe, so try topping this pudding with your favorite fruits.

Strawberries and Cream Chia Pudding

Prep time: 10 min • **Yield:** 3 servings

Ingredients	*Directions*
1 cup strawberries, plus extra for garnish	*1* Remove the green stems from the strawberries and wash.
1 vanilla bean pod	*2* Split the vanilla pod in half lengthways and scrape out the seeds.
2 cups coconut milk (from a carton)	
4 tablespoons honey	*3* In a blender, combine the strawberries, scraped vanilla beans, coconut milk, honey, and lime zest and blend until well combined.
Zest of 1 lime	
4 tablespoons whole chia seeds, plus extra for garnish	*4* In a large bowl, add the strawberry mixture and the chia and whisk thoroughly.
Pepper, to taste (optional)	
	5 Add in a little pepper (if desired).
	6 Let this mixture stand for 10 minutes and whisk again.
	7 Divide the mixture between 3 serving bowls and cover with plastic wrap.
	8 Leave the bowls in the refrigerator for at least 4 hours, but ideally overnight.
	9 Stir the puddings before serving and garnish with extra strawberries and a little sprinkle of whole chia seeds.

Per serving: Calories 201 (From Fat 67); Fat 8g (Saturated 3g); Cholesterol 0mg; Sodium 14mg; Carbohydrate 35g (Dietary Fiber 7g); Protein 3g.

Note: This pudding recipe will keep covered in the refrigerator for up to 5 days, so if you want to make a larger batch for the whole family to enjoy throughout the week, simply double or triple the ingredients.

Vary It! You can substitute any sweetener you like — such as stevia, maple syrup, or agave — for the honey.

Vary It! If strawberries aren't in season or you're not a fan, use different fruits. Try using a ripe mango if they're in season. Peel the mango and cut it lengthways on either side of the stone. This enables you to get at the soft fruit easily with a knife. Remove all the soft fruit you can, and use in place of the strawberries in this recipe.

Espresso Chia Pudding

Prep time: 10 min • **Yield:** 4 servings

Ingredients	Directions
2 cups unsweetened soymilk	*1* In a blender, combine the soymilk, banana, dates, salt, vanilla extract, and espresso powder and blend until smooth.
1 medium ripe banana	
2 Medjool dates, pitted	
¼ teaspoon salt	*2* In a large bowl, add the espresso mixture and the chia, and whisk thoroughly. Let this mixture stand for 10 minutes and whisk again.
½ teaspoon vanilla extract	
1 tablespoon instant espresso powder	
4 tablespoons whole chia seeds	*3* Divide the mixture between 4 serving bowls and cover with plastic wrap. Leave the bowls in the refrigerator for at least 4 hours, but ideally overnight. Stir before serving.

Per serving: Calories 186 (From Fat 49); Fat 6g (Saturated 1g); Cholesterol 0mg; Sodium 210mg; Carbohydrate 30g (Dietary Fiber 6g); Protein 6g.

Vary It! You can use 1 cup of very strong coffee and 1 cup of soymilk in exchange for the 2 cups of soymilk and the espresso powder in this recipe.

How to make good coffee

Not all coffee is created equal. If you want to make the best coffee possible, follow these tips:

✔ Start with fresh coffee beans. Keep the beans fresh in an airtight container. Then, when you're ready to use them, grind the beans yourself (as opposed to buying already ground coffee).

✔ Use high-quality coffee filters — it's worth paying a little extra for a filter that won't break down easily.

✔ Don't skimp on the coffee — use plenty. There's nothing worse than a watery, weak coffee, so if the coffee machine manufacturer suggests an amount, either follow that suggestion or add a bit extra. When you play around a little with the amount, you'll soon learn how much coffee to use to get it to your liking.

✔ Brew the coffee as close to 200 degrees as possible — look at your coffee machine instructions to learn what temperature your machine brews at, or use a thermometer to gauge the temperature.

✔ Keep your coffeemaker and grinder clean.

If you follow these simple steps, you'll get a great cup of coffee every time!

Pumpkin Pie Chia Pudding

Prep time: 10 min • **Yield:** 2 servings

Ingredients	Directions
1 cup pumpkin puree 1½ cups vanilla-flavored coconut milk (from a carton) 1 tablespoon pure maple syrup ½ teaspoon ground cinnamon ¼ teaspoon ground ginger A little grated nutmeg 4 tablespoons whole chia seeds 1 tablespoon desiccated coconut, for garnish	**1** In a large bowl, add the pumpkin puree, coconut milk, maple syrup, cinnamon, ginger, and nutmeg; mix well until all the ingredients are thoroughly combined. **2** Add the chia and stir well. **3** Let this mixture stand for 10 minutes and stir again. **4** Divide the mixture between 2 serving bowls and cover with plastic wrap. **5** Let the bowls sit in the refrigerator for at least 4 hours, but ideally overnight. **6** Stir the puddings before serving, and divide the desiccated coconut between the 2 bowls as a garnish.

Per serving: Calories 253 (From Fat 111); Fat 12g (Saturated 6g); Cholesterol 0mg; Sodium 48mg; Carbohydrate 32g (Dietary Fiber 13g); Protein 6g.

Blueberry Yogurt Chia Parfait

Prep time: 30 min • **Yield:** 4 servings

Ingredients	Directions
2 cups 2 percent milk	**1** In a large bowl, combine the milk, 1 cup of the Greek yogurt, the vanilla extract, and the honey.
2 cups plain Greek yogurt	
¼ teaspoon vanilla extract	**2** Stir in ⅓ cup of the chia seeds.
1 tablespoon honey	
½ cup whole chia seeds	**3** Blend well with a spoon and let this mixture sit in the refrigerator for 20 minutes, stirring occasionally.
1 cup granola	
½ cup fresh blueberries	**4** When the mixture has become thicker, with a gelatinous consistency, divide it evenly between 4 tumbler-size glasses.
½ cup fresh raspberries	
	5 Put ¼ cup of granola into each glass, on top of the chia, milk, and yogurt mixture.
	6 Spoon the remaining Greek yogurt evenly between the glasses, placing the yogurt on top of the granola.
	7 Add some blueberries and raspberries to each glass, and sprinkle the remaining chia seeds on top.

Per serving: Calories 373 (From Fat 113); Fat 13g (Saturated 4g); Cholesterol 16mg; Sodium 110mg; Carbohydrate 47g (Dietary Fiber 10g); Protein 22g.

Note: These parfaits are best eaten immediately, because the chia mixture may soften the granola.

Vary It! You can substitute your favorite non-dairy milk for the milk in this recipe. Try the recipe for homemade almond milk in the "Nutty nut milks" sidebar, earlier in this chapter.

Tip: You can use store-bought granola in this recipe, but they're often very high in sugar so try making your own granola instead. Check out the Classic Granola recipe, earlier in this chapter.

Vary It! You can make this recipe using any fruits that are in season. Try sliced peaches, apples, or oranges, or opt for whatever is fresh and looks good.

Fruit and Nut Yogurt Twist

Prep time: 15 min • **Yield:** 4 servings

Ingredients	Directions
2 medium peaches	**1** Slice the peaches in half, remove the stones, and chop the peaches into small pieces, leaving the skin on.
2 kiwifruits	**2** Peel and slice the kiwifruits.
½ cup raspberries	
½ cup blueberries	**3** In a medium bowl, add the peaches and kiwifruits, and stir to mix together.
½ cup strawberries	
1 tablespoon pistachios	**4** Wash the raspberries and blueberries and add to the peach mixture.
1 tablespoon pecans	
2 tablespoons whole chia seeds	**5** Wash the strawberries and cut into quarters; add to the fruit mixture, stirring well.
4 cups plain Greek yogurt	**6** Chop the pistachios and pecans.
2 tablespoons honey	**7** In a small bowl, mix the pistachios, pecans, and chia.
	8 In each of 4 serving glasses, put one spoonful of the fruit mixture.
	9 In each glass, put a small spoonful of yogurt over the fruit and sprinkle with a little of the nut mixture.
	10 Repeat this layering until all the fruit, nuts, and yogurt are gone, making sure to finish the top layer with the nut mixture.
	11 Drizzle honey over each serving.

Per serving: Calories 328 (From Fat 79); Fat 9g (Saturated 3g); Cholesterol 13mg; Sodium 103mg; Carbohydrate 40g (Dietary Fiber 5g); Protein 26g.

Note: This yogurt mix is best eaten immediately.

Vary It! You can replace any of the nuts with varieties that you enjoy more, such as walnuts, Brazil nuts, hazelnuts, and so on.

Mango Coulis Chia Pudding

Prep time: 15 min • **Yield:** 2 servings

Ingredients	Directions
2 cups coconut milk **1 tablespoon pure maple syrup** **4 tablespoons whole chia seeds, plus extra for garnish** **1 medium ripe mango** **1 tablespoon confectioner's sugar** **3 tablespoons lemon juice** **1 tablespoon water**	**1** In a large bowl, combine the coconut milk, maple syrup, and chia. **2** Whisk until the syrup is well combined. **3** Leave this mixture to set for 10 minutes and whisk again. **4** Divide the mixture between 4 serving glasses, cover, and refrigerate overnight. **5** About an hour before serving, peel the mango, remove the stone, and chop roughly. **6** In a blender, combine the chopped mango, sugar, lemon juice, and water. **7** Blend until smooth, strain through a sieve, and refrigerate the liquid part for at least 30 minutes. **8** Remove the chia pudding mixture from the refrigerator after leaving to set overnight. **9** Divide the mango coulis evenly between the 4 servings of chia pudding. Garnish with whole chia seeds.

Per serving: Calories 294 (From Fat 105); Fat 12g (Saturated 5g); Cholesterol 0mg; Sodium 22mg; Carbohydrate 48g (Dietary Fiber 11g); Protein 5g.

Tip: This pudding can be served as a pretty dessert. Simply slide a butter knife around the edges of the pudding and wiggle it out of the glass into a small bowl.

Note: The pudding will keep fresh in the fridge for 3 days, and the mango coulis will keep fresh for at least 3 days if kept separately. Don't combine the two until you're ready to serve.

Chapter 7

Taking Your Time in the Morning: Cooked Breakfasts

In This Chapter

▶ Cooking perfect eggs every time

▶ Choosing between healthy and traditional pancakes and waffles

▶ Making your mouth water with morning meats

*W*e're all for quick, easy, and nutritious breakfasts, but on the weekends or over holidays, nothing is better than relaxing in the mornings over a warm breakfast. And there's no reason chia seeds can't be part of the ritual. By using chia seeds to boost the nutritional value of your breakfast, you're strengthening your body's defense system so it can handle whatever the day throws at you.

Eggs: Scrambled, Poached, Omelets, and More

Eggs are a nutritious source of quality protein with plenty of vitamins and minerals that are essential for good health. They're inexpensive, easy to cook, and so versatile that you can make many meals based around eggs. Eggs are an especially great breakfast food because they can be cooked alone or added to other foods to create pancakes, omelets, and more, providing your body with some of the nutrients you need throughout the day. Although in the past, there was some concern about the fat contained in eggs, it's now widely accepted that an egg a day is okay — and recommended for good nutrition.

Boiled, Poached, or Fried Eggs

Prep time: 10 min • **Cook time:** 10 min • **Yield:** 1 serving

Ingredients	Directions
2 eggs 1 teaspoon whole chia seeds 2 to 3 tablespoons olive oil (for the fried eggs)	**1** To make boiled eggs, fill a small saucepan with water and bring it to a fast boil. Using a slotted spoon, slowly add the eggs to the saucepan. For soft-boiled eggs, boil the eggs in water for 5 minutes; for medium-cooked eggs, 7½ minutes; for hard-boiled eggs, 10 minutes. To serve your eggs, crack open the eggs and add the chia seeds.
	2 To make poached eggs, fill a wide saucepan with water and a pinch of salt and bring to a boil over medium heat. When the water is softly simmering, gently crack the eggs into the swirling water. For a soft-poached egg, cook for around 2 minutes; for a firm egg, 4 minutes. Remove the eggs from the water with a slotted spoon and dab off excess water with paper towel. Sprinkle with chia seeds before serving.
	3 To make fried eggs, in a medium frying pan, add the olive oil and slowly crack the eggs onto the pan over medium to low heat. As the oil gets hotter, the eggs will start to change color; when they turn white, spoon some of the hot oil back over the yolks of the eggs. If the oil starts to spit, turn down the heat. When they are cooked to your liking, take the pan off the heat and remove the eggs with a slotted spoon. Dab the eggs with paper towel to remove any excess oil and sprinkle the chia seeds over the eggs before serving.

Per serving (boiled and poached): Calories 160 (From Fat 95); Fat 11g (Saturated 3g); Cholesterol 372mg; Sodium 142mg; Carbohydrate 2g (Dietary Fiber 0g); Protein 13g.

Per serving (fried): Calories 398 (From Fat 334); Fat 38g (Saturated 7g); Cholesterol 372mg; Sodium 143mg; Carbohydrate 2g (Dietary Fiber 1g); Protein 13g.

Chia Seed Scrambled Eggs

Prep time: 10 min • **Cook time:** 10 min • **Yield:** 2 servings

Ingredients	Directions
4 eggs 4 tablespoons milk 1 teaspoon milled chia seeds Pinch of salt Pepper, to taste 1 heaping teaspoon butter	**1** In a large bowl, break the eggs and add the milk, chia, salt, and pepper. **2** Whisk the mixture until the whites and yolks are well mixed. **3** In a medium saucepan, place the butter and add the egg mixture. **4** Stir continuously over low heat using a flat-bottomed wooden spatula until the butter has melted and the eggs are soft and creamy. **5** Remove from the heat and stir through again before serving.

Per serving: Calories 184 (From Fat 114); Fat 13g (Saturated 5g); Cholesterol 380mg; Sodium 225mg; Carbohydrate 3g (Dietary Fiber 0g); Protein 14g.

How to tell if eggs are fresh

When you use fresh eggs, the end result of your recipes will be so much better. But how do you know if your eggs are fresh? Fill a bowl with cold water, and gently drop the egg into the bowl. Look at what the egg does.

If it sinks to the bottom of the bowl and lies flat on its side, the egg is very fresh. *If it sinks to the bottom of the bowl but tilts upward slightly,* the egg is about a week old. *If it sinks to the bottom of the bowl but stands straight up,* the egg is several weeks old and going bad. *If the egg floats to the surface, the egg is bad.* Don't eat it.

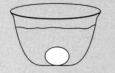

Very fresh

About 1 week old

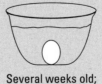

Several weeks old;
going bad

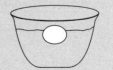

Bad;
do not eat

Deviled Chia Eggs

Prep time: 10 min • **Cook time:** 10 min • **Yield:** 6 servings

Ingredients	Directions
6 eggs	**1** Fill a medium saucepan with water and bring to a boil.
3 tablespoons mayonnaise	**2** Using a slotted spoon, slowly spoon the eggs into the water, and boil for 10 minutes.
1 teaspoon chopped parsley	**3** Drain the water from the saucepan of eggs and fill with cold water, allowing the eggs to cool down.
¼ teaspoon ground mustard	
¼ teaspoon salt	**4** When the eggs are cool to the touch, roll them softly along the countertop, cracking the shells. (This makes it much easier to remove the shells.) Peel all the shells off the eggs and rinse with cold water.
1 tablespoon whole chia seeds	
Sprinkle of paprika	**5** Slice the eggs in half lengthwise, and remove the yolks; place the yolks in a small bowl.
	6 Mash the yolks using a fork, and add the mayonnaise, parsley, mustard, salt, and chia, mixing well.
	7 Spoon the mixture back into the egg whites where the yolks had been.
	8 Sprinkle with paprika, and refrigerate for at least 1 hour or until ready to serve.

Per serving: Calories 127 (From Fat 94); Fat 11g (Saturated 2g); Cholesterol 189mg; Sodium 217mg; Carbohydrate 1g (Dietary Fiber 1g); Protein 7g.

Vary It! If you like spicy foods, try adding 1 teaspoon of cayenne pepper to the egg yolk mixture and mix thoroughly before transferring back to the egg whites.

Baked Chia Eggs with Smoked Haddock

Prep time: 10 min • **Cook time:** 20 min • **Yield:** 6 servings

Ingredients	Directions
½ **cup heavy cream**	**1** Preheat the oven to 350 degrees.
6 tablespoons chopped smoked haddock	**2** In a small saucepan over medium heat, bring the cream to a boil and then add the haddock.
2 tablespoons whole chia seeds	**3** Turn down the heat and gently simmer the haddock for 5 minutes, ensuring that it's cooked through.
2 tablespoons chopped parsley	**4** Using a 6-cup muffin tin, lightly spray each section with some nonstick cooking spray.
6 eggs	**5** Divide the cream and haddock mixture between the 6 cups.
Salt and pepper, to taste	**6** Sprinkle the chia and parsley evenly over the haddock and cream mixture.
	7 Crack 1 egg on top of each haddock-and-cream mixture and season with salt and pepper.
	8 Bake for about 12 minutes for a soft egg, 15 minutes for a medium egg, and 20 minutes for a hard egg.
	9 Remove the eggs from the muffin tin with a spoon and serve immediately.

Per serving: Calories 169 (From Fat 120); Fat 13g (Saturated 6g); Cholesterol 221mg; Sodium 249mg; Carbohydrate 3g (Dietary Fiber 1g); Protein 10g.

Tip: If you don't have a large muffin tin, use small ramekin dishes or even some ovenproof mugs to bake your eggs.

Vary It! Try adding cayenne pepper and cream to the bottom of the muffin tin before adding the egg, or try cheese and cream. You can change things up to vary the flavors — just add whatever ingredients you want to try before you crack the eggs into the muffin tin.

Hearty Chia Breakfast Eggs

Prep time: 5 min • **Cook time:** 10–12 min • **Yield:** 2 servings

Ingredients	Directions
4 eggs	**1** In a medium bowl, crack the eggs, add the milk, and whisk until well mixed.
2 tablespoons milk	
1 tablespoon whole chia seeds (preferably white)	**2** Add the chia to the mixture and stir well. Set aside.
1 tablespoon olive oil	**3** In a small frying pan, heat the olive oil over medium heat and add the onion.
½ small onion, finely chopped	
¼ cup mushrooms	**4** Cook until the onion becomes clear in color.
¼ cup diced bacon	**5** Add the mushrooms and bacon. Cook until the mushrooms are cooked through and slightly browned.
¼ cup baby spinach	
Salt and pepper, to taste	
1 ripe tomato	**6** Turn down the heat and add the chia and egg mixture to the pan.
	7 Cook the mixture until set, stirring continuously using a flat-bottomed wooden spoon.
	8 Add the spinach and stir through the mixture until the leaves are wilted.
	9 Season with salt and pepper.
	10 Cut the tomato into quarters.
	11 Divide the hearty egg mixture between 2 serving plates and add 2 quarter pieces of the tomato alongside each portion.

Per serving: Calories 343 (From Fat 220); Fat 25g (Saturated 7g); Cholesterol 389mg; Sodium 471mg; Carbohydrate 10g (Dietary Fiber 3g); Protein 20g.

Vary It! These eggs are great topped with extra chia seeds to add even more nutrients to your breakfast. You can use whatever vegetables you have in your fridge, so experiment! For example, you might want to try bell peppers, scallions, or zucchini.

Chia Seed Omelet with Asparagus

Prep time: 5 min • **Cook time:** 6–8 min • **Yield:** 1 serving

Ingredients	Directions
1 tablespoon milled chia seeds 2 tablespoons water 2 eggs 4 asparagus spears 1 teaspoon butter 1 teaspoon olive oil Salt and pepper, to taste	**1** In a small bowl, soak the chia seeds in the water and stir well. Leave the mixture to sit for 20 minutes or more, stirring occasionally. This will make a very thick gel. Crack the eggs into this mixture and whisk well. **2** Put the asparagus spears into a steamer basket and cover with a lid. Bring a medium saucepan of water to a boil over high heat and put the steamer basket of asparagus over the pot of water. Steam the asparagus for 2 minutes and remove from the heat. **3** In a nonstick medium frying pan, melt the butter over medium heat. Add the olive oil to prevent the butter from burning and heat gently. **4** Whisk the egg and milled chia seed mixture again to prevent the seeds from clumping. Pour the mixture into the frying pan and heat gently, covering with a lid. **5** Just before the top of the omelet cooks completely, add the asparagus spears and replace the lid. Push in the edges of the omelet to the center to help everything cook evenly. Cook until the top of the omelet is set and only wobbles a small bit. Using a lid will help the top set faster while preventing the bottom from burning. **6** Season with salt and pepper. Fold over the omelet to serve.

Per serving: Calories 260 (From Fat 177); Fat 20g (Saturated 6g); Cholesterol 382mg; Sodium 292mg; Carbohydrate 6g (Dietary Fiber 3g); Protein 15g.

Chia Seed French Toast with Bacon

Prep time: 5 min • **Cook time:** 10 min • **Yield:** 2 servings

Ingredients	Directions
2 eggs	**1** In a small bowl, crack the eggs and add the chia seeds and milk. Whisk well and season with salt and pepper.
1 tablespoon milled chia seeds	
1 tablespoon milk	**2** Dip the bread into the egg mixture, allowing it to soak up the liquid.
Salt and pepper, to taste	
2 slices bread	**3** In a large nonstick frying pan, heat the butter and oil.
1 teaspoon butter	
1 tablespoon olive oil	**4** Add the soaked bread to the frying pan and cook over low heat until gently browned.
4 strips bacon	
2 tablespoons pure maple syrup	**5** Meanwhile, in a separate medium frying pan, fry the bacon in its own fat until crisp.
	6 Remove the cooked bread from the heat and put each slice onto serving plates.
	7 Add 2 strips of bacon to each slice of bread and drizzle with maple syrup to serve.

Per serving: Calories 371 (From Fat 201); Fat 23g (Saturated 7g); Cholesterol 210mg; Sodium 482mg; Carbohydrate 27g (Dietary Fiber 2g); Protein 15g.

Vary It! You can serve this French toast sweeter with sugar and lemon. Just add some confectioner's sugar and lemon after the toast is cooked and sprinkle extra whole chia seeds on top for extra nutrients.

Vary It! Although bacon and maple syrup is a classic combination, there are infinite ways to serve French toast. Try adding yogurt and fresh fruits for a different taste. If it's a very special occasion, try vanilla ice cream and chocolate sauce.

Pancakes and Waffles

Pancakes and waffles are always such a treat and a lovely weekend breakfast to enjoy with the whole family. Kids love them, and adding the extra toppings and experimenting with what goes well with which ingredients is all part of the fun of lazy mornings where family time is precious. Chia can play a part in these not-so-healthy recipes by adding to the nutrient value of your treats. So, if you're going to splurge and make pancakes with whole milk and add all the guilt-laden extras like syrup and chocolate, go ahead and add some chia seeds and lessen the guilt.

Although the common perception of pancakes and waffles is the unhealthy, sugar-laden, high-carbohydrate kind, there is an alternative. With so many different flours and sugar substitutes available today, you can have pancakes or waffles and not go the unhealthy route. In this section, we give you healthy alternative pancake and waffle recipes made with chia seeds to make it an ultimate healthy choice.

The history of pancakes

Pancakes have a long history. Even the word *pancake* appeared in print as early as 1430, and there is evidence to suggest that people in Neolithic times ate pancakes. They would have ground down some wheat, mixed it with goat's milk and bird's egg, and cooked the batter on a heated rock over the campfire. They had no need for frying pans or waffle irons.

Maybe because of this ancient background, pancakes are often associated with rituals such as Shrove Tuesday, often referred to as Pancake Day, where Catholics around the world eat as many pancakes as possible. Medieval pancakes were often made using barley or rye and were quite heavy in comparison to today's fluffy varieties.

Pancakes have evolved to become a staple American breakfast food because they're easy to make and delicious. They're the ultimate crowd pleaser.

Pancakes with Chia Seeds

Prep time: 10 min • **Cook time:** 20 min • **Yield:** 4 servings

Ingredients	Directions
1 cup flour	*1* Preheat the oven to 200 degrees.
1 tablespoon baking powder	
1 tablespoon sugar	*2* In a large bowl, combine the flour, baking powder, sugar, salt, and chia, and mix well.
Pinch of salt	
4 tablespoons whole chia seeds	*3* Make a well in the center of the dry ingredients, and beat in the eggs, butter, and milk. If you have a pouring jug, transfer the mixture to the jug for easier pouring.
2 eggs, beaten	
2 tablespoons butter, melted and cooled, plus extra for frying	*4* In a large frying pan over medium heat, heat some butter.
1 cup milk	*5* Pour the batter onto the hot frying pan to make your pancakes. You should be able to fit 2 or 3 pancakes on a large frying pan.
	6 Cook until the surface of the pancakes has some bubbles and a few have burst, around 1 to 2 minutes.
	7 Flip the pancakes carefully with a spatula and cook the other side, another 1 to 2 minutes.
	8 Transfer the pancakes to a baking sheet and keep them warm in the oven.
	9 Continue cooking your pancakes with more butter and the remaining batter. You should be able to make 8 to 10 pancakes from this amount of batter.

Per serving: Calories 301 (From Fat 122); Fat 14g (Saturated 6g); Cholesterol 114mg; Sodium 400mg; Carbohydrate 35g (Dietary Fiber 5g); Protein 10g.

Tip: Add your favorite toppings — such as pure maple syrup, confectioner's sugar, jam, honey, chocolate syrup, whipped cream, or whatever else you like. You can also try adding healthier toppings such as chopped fruits, nut butters, and natural sugar alternatives (like stevia), with lemon or lime juice. Adding extra chia seeds as a topping will increase the nutrient value further, so go ahead and use more chia!

Alternative Pancakes

Prep time: 10 min • **Cook time:** 20 min • **Yield:** 4 servings

Ingredients	Directions
1 cup whole-grain buckwheat flour	**1** Preheat the oven to 200 degrees.
4 tablespoons quinoa flour	**2** In a large bowl, mix the flours, baking powder, and stevia together.
4 tablespoons coconut flour	
1 tablespoon baking powder	**3** In a blender, blend the almond milk, banana, vanilla, lemon zest, and lemon juice.
4 tablespoons stevia	
2 cups almond milk	**4** Add the blended wet ingredients to the flour mixture and whisk to form a smooth batter.
3 medium ripe bananas, peeled	
1 tablespoon vanilla extract	**5** Stir in the chia seeds. After the chia is fully incorporated, set aside for 10 minutes to allow the seeds to swell and the batter to thicken. Whisk again before cooking and transfer the batter to a pouring jug, if you have one.
Zest of 2 lemons	
Juice of 1 lemon	
4 tablespoon whole chia seeds	
	6 Spray a large frying pan with light cooking spray and place over medium heat.
	7 Pour the batter onto the frying pan to make your pancakes. You should be able to fit 2 or 3 pancakes on a large pan. Cook until the surface of the pancakes has some bubbles and a few have burst, around 1 to 2 minutes. Flip carefully with a spatula and cook the other side, another 1 to 2 minutes.
	8 Transfer the pancakes to a baking sheet and keep them warm in the oven.
	9 Continue cooking your pancakes with more light cooking spray and the remaining batter. You should be able to make 12 to 14 pancakes from this amount of batter.

Per serving: Calories 319 (From Fat 68); Fat 8g (Saturated 2g); Cholesterol 0mg; Sodium 393mg; Carbohydrate 55g (Dietary Fiber 15g); Protein 9g.

Chia Seed Waffles

Prep time: 10 min • **Cook time:** 20 min • **Yield:** 6 servings

Ingredients	Directions
6 eggs	*1* Preheat a waffle iron to high heat.
⅓ cup melted butter	
1 cup milk	*2* In a large bowl, beat together the eggs, butter, milk, and vanilla.
1 teaspoon vanilla extract	
⅓ cup sugar	*3* In a separate medium bowl, mix together the sugar, flour, salt, baking powder, and chia.
2 cups flour	
½ teaspoon salt	*4* Add the dry ingredients to the wet and mix thoroughly using a wire whisk.
1 tablespoon baking powder	
4 tablespoons whole chia seeds	*5* Transfer the batter to a pouring jug, if you have one, and pour the batter onto the waffle iron. This recipe makes around 6 large waffles, depending on the size of your waffle iron.
12 tablespoons pure maple syrup	
2 tablespoons confectioner's sugar	*6* Close the lid of the waffle iron and wait around 4 minutes or until the indicator shows that the waffles are ready.
1 cup strawberries	*7* Place a waffle on each of 6 serving plates.
6 tablespoons sweetened whipped cream	*8* Drizzle each plate with maple syrup and sprinkle the confectioner's sugar evenly among the servings.
2 tablespoons whole chia seeds, for garnish	*9* Divide the strawberries evenly among the plates.
	10 Add a tablespoon of sweetened whipped cream to each serving.
	11 Garnish with chia.

Per serving: Calories 578 (From Fat 198); Fat 22g (Saturated 11g); Cholesterol 225mg; Sodium 493mg; Carbohydrate 82g (Dietary Fiber 5g); Protein 14g.

Vary It! To make this dish a little healthier, swap the toppings for a mixture of fresh fruits and yogurt.

Healthy Whole-Wheat Waffles

Prep time: 10 min • **Cook time:** 20 min • **Yield:** 6 servings

Ingredients	Directions
2 medium ripe bananas	*1* Preheat a waffle iron to high heat.
½ cup unsweetened applesauce	*2* In a large bowl, mash the bananas with a fork until they make a smooth paste. Add the applesauce and eggs and whisk together. Add the buttermilk to the mixture and continue to whisk to combine thoroughly.
2 eggs	
1½ cups buttermilk	
1 cup rolled oats, roughly chopped	*3* In a separate medium bowl, mix together the oats, flour, chia, baking powder, salt, vanilla sugar, and cinnamon. Stir to ensure they're mixed well.
1 cup whole-wheat flour	
4 tablespoons whole chia seeds	*4* Add the dry ingredients to the wet and mix thoroughly using a wire whisk.
1 tablespoon baking powder	
½ teaspoon salt	*5* Transfer the batter to a pouring jug, if you have one, and pour the batter onto the waffle iron. This recipe will make around 6 large waffles, depending on the size of your waffle iron.
1 teaspoon vanilla sugar	
½ teaspoon cinnamon	
1 cup plain Greek yogurt	
1 cup fresh blueberries	*6* Close the lid of the waffle iron and wait around 4 minutes or until the indicator shows that they're ready.
6 tablespoons honey	
1 tablespoon whole chia seeds, for garnish	*7* Place a waffle on each of 6 serving plates. Spoon the yogurt evenly among the plates, top with blueberries, and drizzle with honey. Top with extra chia seeds for garnish.

Per serving: Calories 363 (From Fat 66); Fat 7g (Saturated 2g); Cholesterol 67mg; Sodium 501mg; Carbohydrate 65g (Dietary Fiber 9g); Protein 14g.

Tip: If you find that your waffles tend to stick to the waffle iron a little, spray the iron with light cooking oil before use.

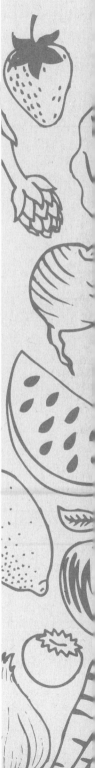

Morning Meats to Make Your Mouth Water

Many cultures around the world enjoy meat in the mornings. Sometimes it's simply cold meats served with fresh breads, as is the norm in many European countries. Other times, it's the not-so-healthy fried meats that you see served at hotel breakfast buffets.

Having meat in the morning gives your body some much-needed protein, but be sure to choose wisely. Try to select meats that are lower in saturated fat and salt and don't have too many other ingredients. If you're buying bacon products, make sure they have a high percentage of pork in them and aren't made up of too many fillers.

If you're buying fresh meat, choose cuts that have visibly less fat on them and ask your butcher where he sources his meat. All sources of meat should be able to be traced back to the farm it was produced on, so if you can't find out this information, choose a different butcher.

This chapter gives you a few examples of how different cultures use meats in the mornings, but we've made the recipes a little healthier and more heart healthy by changing the cooking methods, choosing healthier ingredients, and adding chia seeds.

Irish Breakfast Fry-up

Prep time: 15 min • **Cook time:** 15 min • **Yield:** 2 servings

Ingredients	*Directions*
2 ripe tomatoes	*1* Preheat the broiler to high and put a wire rack over a baking tray. Halve the tomatoes and put them on the wire rack, cut side up. Trim the stalks from the mushrooms and put them on the wire rack, stalk side up. Run a knife lengthwise down the middle of the sausages, without cutting through; then open them up, flatten them down, and put them on the wire rack. Season the tomatoes and mushrooms with salt and pepper and spray lightly with light cooking spray.
2 large mushrooms	
2 strips bacon	
2 small breakfast sausages	
Salt and pepper, to taste	
One 8-ounce can baked beans	*2* Remove the fat from the bacon. Set aside.
2 tablespoons whole chia seeds	*3* Place the tray under the broiler for 5 minutes.
4 slices whole-grain bread	*4* Fill a medium saucepan with water and bring to a boil over high heat.
2 eggs	*5* After 5 minutes, add the bacon to the wire rack and turn the sausages. Cook for another 5 minutes, until the bacon is golden and crispy.
	6 Meanwhile, in a small saucepan, place the beans and heat over medium heat. After the beans are heated, remove them from the heat, add the chia, and stir well.
	7 Put the bread into the toaster.
	8 Crack the eggs into the pan of simmering water and poach for 3 minutes. Remove the eggs from the water with a slotted spoon and dab dry with paper towels.
	9 Divide everything between 2 plates. Each serving gets 2 slices of toast, 2 halves of tomato, 1 mushroom, 1 sausage, 2 strips of bacon, 1 egg, and a good-size serving of baked beans.

Per serving: Calories 583 (From Fat 239); Fat 27g (Saturated 7g); Cholesterol 209mg; Sodium 987mg; Carbohydrate 59g (Dietary Fiber 13g); Protein 30g.

Vietnamese Beef Breakfast Soup

Prep time: 15 min • **Cook time:** 20 min • **Yield:** 4 servings

Ingredients	Directions
1 thumb-size piece fresh ginger, peeled and finely sliced	*1* In a large saucepan, bring the beef broth to a boil and add the ginger, star anise, and cinnamon. Reduce the heat and simmer for 15 minutes.
6 cups beef broth	
2 whole star anise	
1 cinnamon stick	*2* Meanwhile, with a very sharp knife, cut the sirloin across the grain into very thin slices.
½ pound beef sirloin	
3 ounces dried flat rice noodles	*3* In a large bowl, soak the noodles in hot water and cover for 15 minutes, or until softened and pliable. Drain the noodles into a colander.
¼ cup fish sauce	
Pepper, to taste	*4* In a medium saucepan, bring salted water to a boil, add the noodles, and cook for around 1 minute. Drain the noodles again and set aside.
1 cup fresh bean sprouts, rinsed and drained	
⅓ cup scallions, finely chopped	*5* Remove the cinnamon stick and star anise from the broth. Add the fish sauce, pepper, beef, and bean sprouts.
¼ cup fresh cilantro sprigs, finely chopped	*6* Continue to cook for less than a minute or until the beef begins to change color; skim any excess froth from the top of the soup.
1 bird's eye red or green chili, finely sliced	
½ cup fresh basil leaves	*7* In 4 deep serving dishes, divide the noodles evenly. Ladle the soup evenly between the dishes and sprinkle the scallions, cilantro, chili, basil, and chia over each of the servings.
4 tablespoons whole chia seeds	
4 lime wedges, for garnish	*8* Serve immediately and garnish each portion of soup with a wedge of lime.

Per serving: Calories 281 (From Fat 87); Fat 10g (Saturated 2g); Cholesterol 37mg; Sodium 2,798mg; Carbohydrate 26g (Dietary Fiber 6g); Protein 24g.

Homemade Sausage Breakfast Sandwiches

Prep time: 15 min • **Cook time:** 20 min • **Yield:** 8 servings

Ingredients	Directions
4 tablespoons whole chia seeds	**1** In a large bowl, combine the chia, sage, thyme, salt, and pepper.
2 teaspoons dried sage	
¼ teaspoon dried thyme	**2** Add the onion, garlic, pork, and water.
2 teaspoons salt	**3** Use your hands to thoroughly combine all the ingredients, squashing everything together.
1 teaspoon pepper	
½ small onion, minced	**4** Once the ingredients are mixed well and you can see that the chia seeds are evenly dispersed, take a small handful of sausage meat and form it into patties.
1 clove garlic, minced	
2 pounds ground pork	
¼ cup water	**5** Repeat this step until all the meat is gone. You should get around 8 good-size patties from this amount of meat.
2 tablespoons olive oil	
16 slices whole-grain bread	
8 tablespoons butter	**6** In a large frying pan, heat 1 tablespoon of the olive oil and add 4 of the patties to the pan. Cook over medium heat for 5 minutes on each side. Repeat for the remaining patties.
8 tablespoons relish	
	7 Meanwhile, toast the bread. Spread the butter on the toasted bread and add a sausage patty.
	8 Spoon the relish on top of the sausage and cover with another slice of toast to serve the sandwiches.

Per serving: Calories 554 (From Fat 317); Fat 36g (Saturated 15g); Cholesterol 106mg; Sodium 981mg; Carbohydrate 29g (Dietary Fiber 6g); Protein 29g.

Tip: If you're feeding children or not-so-hungry adults, make smaller sausage patties — you'll just get more of them.

Chapter 8

Smoothies and Juices: Nutrition in a Glass

In This Chapter

▶ Following the basic steps to smoothie making

▶ Using chia to add nutrients to the best smoothie recipes

A quick breakfast shouldn't mean missing out on important nutrition to start your day. Even if you're rushing out the door with kids, smoothies and juices are a fantastic way to get the nutrients you need.

In this chapter, we walk you through the basic steps of putting a nutritious breakfast into a glass, quickly and easily. We also discuss the benefits that little changes make to your health such as using fresh or frozen produce and milk alternatives.

Chia Smoothie Basics

Chia gives any smoothie a great nutritional kick and is simple to prepare. You can add chia to a smoothie in two ways:

✔ **Create a chia gel and add it to the smoothie.** This approach softens the seed prior to adding it to the smoothie. To make a chia gel, mix one part chia seeds to six parts water, stir, let sit for a few minutes, and stir again. Leave for ten minutes more, and use as necessary. If the texture of the smoothie made with chia gel is too thick for your taste, just add more water.

✔ **Add ground or milled chia seeds to your smoothie.** You can buy ground or milled chia or just grind the whole seeds yourself in a coffee grinder.

To create any smoothie, follow these five basic steps:

1. **Start with a liquid base.**

   The amount of liquid required will depend on your desired consistency and how many servings you want to make. You can use anything from ½ cup to 3 cups of liquid, but start off with less than you think you need — you can always add more liquid at the end for a thinner consistency.

   You can use any liquid you like, such as water, coconut water, juice, milk, or yogurt. Pay attention to the nutritional value of the liquid you're adding — you could end up adding a lot of sugar to your smoothie without realizing it.

2. **Add fruits and/or vegetables.**

   Choosing which fruits or vegetables to add to your smoothies can be a learning curve — you can put anything into a smoothie, but some foods are very overpowering and you may end up with a flavor that you don't like. Smoothie making is about trial and error, so don't be afraid to experiment.

   Some veggies that work great in a smoothie are carrots, spinach, cucumber, and kale. Fruits that work well are pears, peaches, pineapple, and soft berries.

3. **Add extra flavor and nutrition.**

   Depending on the fruits and vegetables you're using, a bit of sweetness can be added if desired, but make sure to avoid table sugar and artificial sweeteners. Instead, choose natural options such as honey, stevia, or vanilla extract. Some people like adding spices, so give cinnamon or nutmeg a go and see if you like the taste. You can add anything you like to give the smoothie a flavor and nutrient boost, but try to use natural, unprocessed ingredients.

   Chia can be added to every smoothie you make to give it a nutrient kick that your body needs.

4. Consider texture and temperature.

At this stage, you have all the goodness in the smoothie, but if it's too thick or too runny or not the right temperature, you won't enjoy your smoothie experience.

Ice is a great option for thickening a smoothie and getting it colder. Chia gel is another great thickener. Or try adding an extra banana or some yogurt to change the consistency. *Remember:* Keep experimenting to find what you like.

5. Blend.

Finally, you can blend it all together to make the drink. Initially, pulse the blender to get everything mixed up, and then let the blender liquefy everything until it gets nice and smooth and to your desired consistency. If the smoothie is too thick, just add more liquid. Pour and enjoy.

Here are some final smoothie-making tips:

- ✔ If you're looking for a low-calorie smoothie, stick to water, fruit, and ice.
- ✔ If the blender gets stuck during blending, stop it, open the lid, and shake; then try blending again. If it's still stuck, slowly add liquid.
- ✔ If your smoothie is too sweet, add a pinch of sea salt.
- ✔ If your smoothie is bitter, add a sweet fruit such as a pineapple, a few dates, ripe berries, or overripe banana.
- ✔ Make your smoothies when you're ready to enjoy them. The longer your smoothie sits, the less nutritious it becomes.

For even more smoothie recipes, check out *Juicing & Smoothies For Dummies,* by Pat Crocker (Wiley). *Remember:* You can add chia seeds to any smoothie!

Green Fruit and Veggie Smoothie Combo

Prep time: 10 min • **Yield:** 3 servings

Ingredients	Directions
2 medium apples	**1** Chop the apple and kiwi into smaller pieces, leaving out the apple core.
2 kiwifruits, peeled	
3 tablespoons whole chia seeds	**2** Create a chia gel by mixing the chia and water; set aside.
1⅛ cup water	
1 banana, peeled	**3** In a blender, place all the ingredients, including the chia gel, and pulse to mix. Blend until all the ingredients are liquefied.
⅓ cup spinach	
⅔ cup pineapple juice	
⅓ cup frozen pineapple pieces	
1 cup frozen mango pieces	
2 cups ice	

Per serving: Calories 242 (From Fat 35); Fat 4g (Saturated 0g); Cholesterol 0mg; Sodium 9mg; Carbohydrate 52g (Dietary Fiber 11g); Protein 3g.

Fresh or frozen?

The decision on whether to use fresh or frozen fruits and vegetables has a big impact on the end result of smoothies — it affects the texture and taste. Plus, there's a lot of debate on the nutritional difference between fresh and frozen.

Fresh fruits and vegetables that are harvested locally and arrive at your store having had less chance to lose their nutrients, whereas those that travel farther are picked before they're fully ripe and may not have all the nutrition because they aren't fully developed. Frozen fruits and vegetables are picked at their ripest and frozen quite quickly, retaining their nutrients, which makes them a good option if fresh fruits and vegetables aren't available.

The key is to be aware of where your fresh fruits and vegetables are coming from. If they're sourced locally, you can always freeze them when you buy them, and use as needed.

Standard Protein Smoothie

Prep time: 10 min • **Yield:** 2 servings

Ingredients	Directions
1 cup frozen strawberries 1 banana, peeled 2 tablespoons vanilla protein powder 2 cups almond milk 2 tablespoons milled chia seeds	In a blender, place all the ingredients and blend until smooth.

Per serving: Calories 252 (From Fat 49); Fat 6g (Saturated 0g); Cholesterol 0mg; Sodium 245mg; Carbohydrate 40g (Dietary Fiber 6g); Protein 13g.

Dairy alternatives

Animal milks, such as cow's milk or goat's milk, have been used for centuries as a source of protein, calcium, vitamins, and fat. Today we're seeing more and more nut-based milks, such as almond milk or cashew milk. Nut milks are produced by soaking the nuts in water for hours, blending them, and then straining the mixture through a muslin cloth or nut bag. Nut milks are full of nutrients from the nuts and none of the animal fats found in animal milks.

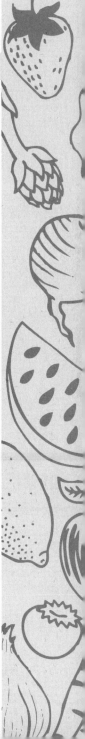

Green Protein Smoothie

Prep time: 10 min • **Yield:** 1 serving

Ingredients	Directions
½ **cup frozen broccoli**	**1** In a blender, place all the ingredients and pulse.
1 cup spinach	
1 cup kale	**2** After the ingredients are well mixed, blend until the desired consistency is attained.
½ **celery stalk**	
1 tablespoon milled chia seeds	
1 cup cold water	
1 cup apple juice	
1 tablespoon vanilla protein powder	

Per serving: Calories 297 (From Fat 30); Fat 3g (Saturated 0g); Cholesterol 0mg; Sodium 209mg; Carbohydrate 56g (Dietary Fiber 8g); Protein 17g.

Vary It! If you don't particularly like broccoli, spinach, or kale, change the green produce to something else. If you have pea protein powder, you can use this instead of the vanilla protein powder to add more green power.

How to eat clean with chia

Chia can help you stick to your clean eating plan. *Eating clean* basically means eating a nutritionally balanced diet but also staying away from processed foods so that your diet is made up of natural foods. Because chia is 100 percent natural, you can get great nutrients from it without compromising your eating clean principles.

To eat clean, stick to the following tips:

✔ Avoid overly processed foods.

✔ Avoid additives and artificial ingredients.

✔ Eat whole foods.

✔ Cut down on sugar.

✔ Cook your own meals.

✔ Use herbs and spices.

Summer Fresh Smoothie

Prep time: 10 min • **Yield:** 2 servings

Ingredients	Directions
2 tablespoons whole chia seeds	*1* Create a chia gel by mixing the chia and water; set aside.
¾ cup water	
2 cups frozen mixed berries	*2* In a blender, add all the ingredients, including the chia gel, and blend until the desired consistency is attained.
½ cup lemon juice	
1 cup apple juice	
1 cup strawberry sorbet	

Per serving: Calories 288 (From Fat 30); Fat 3g (Saturated 0g); Cholesterol 0mg; Sodium 7mg; Carbohydrate 68g (Dietary Fiber 10g); Protein 3g.

Tip: Add ice if you want the smoothie cooler.

Vary It! Add different berries or sorbet to change the flavor to your liking.

The power of berries

Berries are loaded with antioxidants that help fight disease. Raspberries, strawberries, blackberries, and blueberries are delicious to eat and are available in most places so they're a great way to fill up on your antioxidant needs. Even if they aren't in season, frozen berries can be purchased year-round and are just as nutritious. A handful of berries (frozen or fresh) added to a smoothie makes it taste great and gives it a fabulous color. Most important, they add disease-fighting antioxidants. Antioxidants help repair cells from oxidation and help prevent *free radicals* (the disease-causing compounds) from building up and causing harm to your body's cells. Try to include as many antioxidants in your diet as possible. Chia is a great source of antioxidants, but so are berries — if you eat chia and berries every day, you'll be going a long way toward helping to prevent disease.

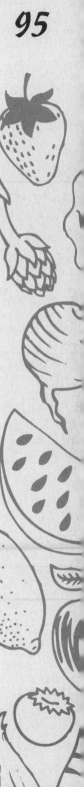

Caribbean Twist Smoothie

Prep time: 10 min • **Yield:** 8 servings

Ingredients	Directions
4 cups coconut water **½ cup lime juice** **¼ cup fresh mint** **6 cups frozen pineapple chunks** **¼ cup milled chia seeds**	In a blender, place all the ingredients and blend until the desired consistency is attained.

Per serving: Calories 103 (From Fat 10); Fat 1g (Saturated 1g); Cholesterol 0mg; Sodium 10mg; Carbohydrate 24g (Dietary Fiber 3g); Protein 1g.

Tip: You may need to divide the ingredients in half and blend in two batches, depending on the size of your blender.

Note: This recipe serves 8 people, so if you're only making it for 2 people, simply divide the ingredients by 4.

Vary It! This smoothie is great at a party, so if it's all adults, go ahead and add some rum! Just be sure to tell people that there's alcohol in there.

The dreaded hangover

If you have a few too many drinks, you can bet you'll feel it the next day. But chia can be your friend when you're nursing a hangover. Typically, you feel hung over because you're completely dehydrated, so when you get up in the morning, drink plenty of water and have some chia seeds — either include them in your breakfast or throw some into a juice and knock it back. This will help your body rehydrate. Plus, the chia seeds will absorb the liquid and hydrate your body slowly throughout the day. Chia seeds also give you the energy you need to get through your day — which is especially important when you're hung over, because even the simplest tasks seem a lot harder.

Healthy Carrot Cardio Smoothie

Prep time: 10 min • **Yield:** 1 serving

Ingredients	*Directions*
2 carrots	*1* Cut the carrots and leek into chunks and put them through a juicer, retaining the juice.
¼ leek	
¼ cup parsley	*2* In a blender, place the juice from the carrots and leeks along with the parsley, carrot juice, chia, and ice and blend until the desired consistency is attained.
1 cup carrot juice	
1 tablespoon ground chia seeds	
½ cup ice cubes	

Per serving: Calories 193 (From Fat 19); Fat 2g (Saturated 0g); Cholesterol 0mg; Sodium 288mg; Carbohydrate 38g (Dietary Fiber 5g); Protein 6g.

Note: Add more ice cubes if the texture is too thick.

Tip: Add vitamin C crystal powder to boost your immunity.

Dieting with chia

Having a healthy body weight is one of the best things you can do for your health. Carrying around excess weight puts pressure on your heart, kidneys, and other organs so ditching the extra weight can improve your health immensely. You can lose weight by eliminating junk food from your diet, eating more plant proteins (such as peas, beans, quinoa, nuts, and, of course, chia seeds), avoiding sugary drinks (including fruit juices) and trans fats, cutting down on alcohol, and controlling portion sizes.

Chia can also help you achieve your weight loss goals. Eat or drink ½ tablespoon of chia seeds mixed with water about 30 minutes before each meal. This will make you feel fuller and encourage you to eat less. Be sure to drink at least eight glasses of water a day when you're consuming chia. Chia is hydrophilic and needs water to do its job.

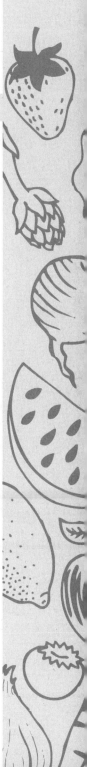

Christmas Nutritious Smoothie

Prep time: 10 min • **Yield:** 1 serving

Ingredients	*Directions*
1 tablespoon whole chia seeds	*1* Create a chia gel by mixing the chia and water; set aside.
6 tablespoons water	
1 banana, peeled	*2* In the blender, place the banana, yogurt, eggnog, and ice and blend until the desired texture is attained.
1 cup nonfat plain Greek yogurt	
1 cup light eggnog	*3* Add the chia gel and blend again.
1 cup ice cubes	
Ground nutmeg, for garnish	*4* Pour the smoothie into a glass, and garnish with nutmeg.

Per serving: Calories 569 (From Fat 122); Fat 14g (Saturated 6g); Cholesterol 111mg; Sodium 254mg; Carbohydrate 80g (Dietary Fiber 7g); Protein 38g.

Vary It! Add 1 ounce of brandy to the smoothie if you're feeling festive.

The Chia Pet: The novelty gift that rocked the '80s

If you watched TV in the 1980s, you know all about Chia Pets. You can probably sing the theme song ("Ch-ch-ch-chia!"). These novelty gifts were big business, and you can still buy them today. Chia Pets come in all different shapes and sizes — one of the latest is a likeness of President Barack Obama. The seeds used to grow grassy "hair" or "fur" on the clay figurines were, indeed, chia seeds. Little did anyone know the great nutrition that those seeds contained. Thankfully, today we know the value of chia and can put it to use nourishing our own bodies instead of the popular clay figures.

By the way, don't eat the chia seeds that came with your Chia Pet. They may grow "hair" or "fur" on your Chia Pet just fine, but they're not suitable for human consumption. Opt for high-quality chia seeds like the kind we refer to in this book instead.

Coffee Smoothie

Prep time: 10 min • **Yield:** 1 serving

Ingredients	Directions
1 tablespoon whole chia seeds 6 tablespoons water	*1* Create a chia gel by mixing the chia and water; set aside.
1 cup coffee ½ cup soymilk	*2* In a blender, place the coffee, soymilk, banana, honey, and ice and blend together.
1 frozen banana, peeled 1 teaspoon manuka honey 6 ice cubes	*3* Add the chia gel to the blender and blend again until the desired consistency is attained.

Per serving: Calories 245 (From Fat 52); Fat 6g (Saturated 1g); Cholesterol 0mg; Sodium 70mg; Carbohydrate 45g (Dietary Fiber 7g); Protein 7g.

Vary It! If you want to indulge, add some of your favorite chocolate powder to this smoothie.

The healing power of manuka honey

Honey has been used since ancient times to treat many conditions, but not until the 19th century were honey's natural antibacterial qualities discovered. Honey can protect against bacterial infection and repair tissue damaged by infection. It also has some anti-inflammatory properties. However, not all honey is created equal — a lot depends on the type of honey and how it's harvested. Manuka honey is said to be the most potent and effective in treating infection. But even the infection-fighting compounds found in manuka honey differ greatly. A scale called the Unique Manuka Factor (UMF) scale measures manuka honey's potency. Manuka honey must have a potency of at least 10 UMF to be considered therapeutic. Then it can be marketed as "active manuka honey."

Remember: No honey is a cure-all, and any serious injury should be treated by a healthcare professional.

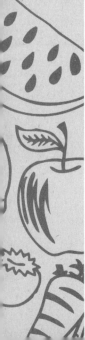

Chocolate Chia Smoothie

Prep time: 10 min • **Yield:** 1 serving

Ingredients	Directions
2 tablespoons whole chia seeds	**1** Create a chia gel by mixing the chia and water; set aside.
¾ cup water	
1 cup 2 percent milk	**2** In a blender, put the milk, cacao powder, cinnamon, maple syrup, and ice and blend together.
1 tablespoon cacao powder	
¼ teaspoon cinnamon	**3** Add the chia gel to the blender and blend again until the desired consistency is attained.
1 teaspoon maple syrup	
1 cup ice cubes	

Per serving: Calories 278 (From Fat 120); Fat 13g (Saturated 5g); Cholesterol 20mg; Sodium 121mg; Carbohydrate 28g (Dietary Fiber 9g); Protein 13g.

The merits of chocolate

Who doesn't love chocolate? Most people like to indulge in a little chocolate from time to time. To make your indulgence just a little bit healthier, choose dark chocolate. Scientists seem to agree that a little indulgent dark chocolate treat every now and again can even be *good* for health! Why? Because of the antioxidants contained in dark chocolate. These antioxidants help fight disease by getting rid of the free radicals caused during oxidation of the cells. These free radicals go on to cause disease, but antioxidants help to prevent their buildup.

Remember: These studies aren't an excuse to go on a chocolate binge. It may be good for you, but you can't live on chocolate alone.

Halloween Fright Night Delight

Prep time: 10 min • **Yield:** 2 servings

Ingredients	Directions
1 tablespoon whole chia seeds	**1** Create a chia gel by mixing the chia and water; set aside.
6 tablespoons water	
1 cup soymilk	**2** In a blender, place the soymilk, protein powder, pumpkin, cinnamon, nutmeg, stevia, and ice and blend together.
1 tablespoon vanilla protein powder	
1 cup canned pumpkin	**3** Add the chia gel to the blender and blend again until the desired consistency is attained.
1 teaspoon cinnamon	
¼ teaspoon ground nutmeg	
1 tablespoon stevia	
6 cubes ice	

Per serving: Calories 122 (From Fat 31); Fat 3g (Saturated 1g); Cholesterol 9mg; Sodium 39mg; Carbohydrate 17g (Dietary Fiber 8g); Protein 9g.

Vary It! You can be bold and use brown sugar in place of the stevia for a real treat.

Using stevia instead of sugar

Recent research is proving that sugar is a huge factor in the rise in obesity levels worldwide. Typical western diets have included more and more sugar since the early 1970s, which coincides with the rise in obesity levels, heart disease, and cancer. Scientists are starting to blame sugar for this epidemic in bad health, so it makes sense that many people are turning to sugar substitutes to satisfy their sugar cravings.

Stevia is a South American herb that has been used as a natural sweetener for centuries. It has no calories and no carbohydrates and is completely natural, so it's a good substitute for sugar and for artificial sweeteners that are manufactured using synthetic ingredients. We're in favor of using as many natural products as possible, so next time you reach for sugar, think about the effects it's having on your body and try stevia instead.

Juicy Juices

Juicing fruits and vegetables is a delicious way to get huge amounts of vitamins and minerals into your system fast. If you have a cough or cold or aren't feeling so well, your body often needs more vitamins and minerals to cope with the extra strain. A freshly squeezed juice can provide these vitamins and minerals quickly.

Many people start their day with a basic green juice to boost their immunity and help fight off infections because of the rich splurge of antioxidants. So, if you feel your immune system could use a pick-me-up, juice some fresh produce, add some chia seeds, and your body will thank you!

Eating in season

It's always good practice to see what fruits and vegetables are grown locally because these are the best ones to use for your smoothies and juices. Locally grown fruits and vegetables that are in season have the most flavor and nutritional value because they haven't had to travel far to get to your grocery store. They're also more affordable.

For the greatest freshness, look for foods that are locally grown and in season. When you know what fruits and vegetables are in season locally, you can choose produce that is affordable and full of nutrients and leads to great-tasting smoothies and juices that your whole family can enjoy.

A great way to find locally grown in-season fruits and vegetables is to visit local farmer's markets. You can also look into community supported agriculture (CSA) programs, which are subscription services where you pay a monthly fee and get fresh fruits and vegetables delivered to your home by a local farm. Use your favorite search engine to find one in your area — just search for your city or town and CSA (for example, "Los Angeles CSA").

Basic Green Power Juice

Prep time: 10 min • **Yield:** 2 servings

Ingredients	Directions
2 Golden Delicious apples	*1* Cut the apples into small pieces that will fit easily through your juicer.
½ pineapple	
2 sticks celery	*2* Peel the skin from the pineapple and cut it into small pieces.
¼ cucumber	
2 cups baby leaf spinach	*3* Put the apples, pineapple, celery, cucumber, spinach, lime, and ginger through the juicer.
Juice of ½ lime	
½-inch piece of fresh ginger, peeled	*4* When your juice is ready, add the milled chia seeds. Stir well before serving immediately.
1 tablespoon milled chia seeds	

Per serving: Calories 234 (From Fat 14); Fat 2g (Saturated 0g); Cholesterol 0mg; Sodium 101mg; Carbohydrate 58g (Dietary Fiber 7g); Protein 3g.

Listen to your mother and eat your greens

When it comes to green vegetables, you really do have the green light to eat as many as you like. Leafy green vegetables and any green vegetables for that matter are a great addition to any diet. They provide valuable nutrients and countless health benefits. They're full of vitamins, minerals, and disease-fighting anti-oxidants. Calcium, vitamin C, and beta-carotene are all found in green vegetables and they all play a role in keeping your body healthy. Green vegetables are also rich in fiber, so they help you maintain a healthy weight by making you feel full. Finally, they provide a slow-release energy that can help control blood sugar levels. So, go ahead and add as many green vegetables to your diet as possible, and encourage your kids to do the same. Sprinkle some chia seeds over your greens for an ultimate nutrient boost. Your body will thank you for it!

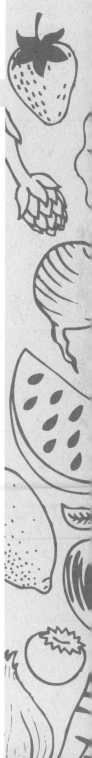

Mango Cranberry Juice

Prep time: 5 min • **Yield:** 1 serving

Ingredients	Directions
1 mango	*1* Peel the mango and remove the center stone.
1 cup fresh cranberries	
1 orange	*2* Put the mango, cranberries, orange, lemon, and ginger through the juicer.
½ lemon, peeled	
½-inch piece fresh ginger	
1 teaspoon manuka honey	*3* Add the honey and chia seeds to the juice. Mix well before serving immediately.
1 tablespoon milled chia seeds	

Per serving: Calories 393 (From Fat 28); Fat 3g (Saturated 0g); Cholesterol 0mg; Sodium 90mg; Carbohydrate 90g (Dietary Fiber 5g); Protein 5g.

Part III
Appetizers, Main Courses, and Something for Everyone

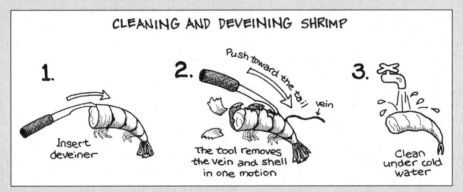

CLEANING AND DEVEINING SHRIMP

1. Insert deveiner

2. Push toward the tail vein
The tool removes the vein and shell in one motion

3. Clean under cold water

Illustration by Elizabeth Kurtzman

In this part . . .

- ✔ Create delicious little bites to enjoy before meals or when you want something to snack on.

- ✔ Expand on your everyday repertoire of main meals and see how easy it is to boost your nutrient intake at every meal.

- ✔ Discover how to get your nutrient requirements when you have to follow a restrictive diet.

- ✔ Make appealing kids' meals with hidden chia so that the little ones will never suspect they're eating healthy.

- ✔ Get the whole family involved in cooking and preparing healthy meals.

Chapter 9

Let's Get This Party Started: Before the Main Course

The food and drinks served before main meals are often calorie dense, nutritionally poor, and rich in saturated fats, so you end up taking in lots of calories before you even touch your meal! This chapter is all about choosing the right foods to serve before dinner so that you don't fall into the trap of ruining your healthy eating intentions before the main course even begins.

In this chapter, we offer recipes for some seriously good salads, healthy soups, and delectable appetizers that will not only make your mouth water but also fuel your body with the right nutrients. We also include a few recipes for chia-infused drinks because food isn't the only thing that you can supercharge with chia — the tiny seeds go really well in all kinds of drinks, too.

Appetizers

Sometimes the best part of a meal is what comes before the main event. Appetizers should be light (so they don't fill you up) but tasty (because what's the point of eating something that isn't?). There's no reason you can't add some highly nutritious chia seeds to these tasty morsels to get your meals off to the right start. The recipes in this section are a mix of vegetarian and fish based, but they're all light enough to have before a main meal.

Spicy Ginger Prawns

Prep time: 10 min • **Cook time:** 10 min • **Yield:** 4 servings

Ingredients	Directions
One 4-inch piece fresh ginger	**1** Peel the ginger and chop into long, thin strips. Try to cut them as thin as you can.
6 cloves garlic	
2 red chilies	**2** Peel the garlic and chop roughly into small pieces. You should get 4 to 5 pieces from each clove.
2 tablespoons olive oil	
24 raw jumbo shrimp, cleaned, peeled, and deveined (see Figure 9-1)	**3** Deseed the chilies and cut lengthways; then chop sideways into small slices.
1 tablespoon whole chia seeds	**4** In a large frying pan, heat the olive oil over medium heat. Add the ginger strips to the frying pan and cook for 2 minutes. Add the shrimp to the frying pan and cook for around 3 minutes, tossing occasionally so they cook well. Add the garlic and chilies to the frying pan and cook for another 2 or 3 minutes.
Pepper, to taste	
Crusty bread, to serve	
	5 Remove from the heat and sprinkle the whole chia seeds over the contents of the pan. Grind black pepper over the pan to serve.
	6 Serve with your favorite crusty bread, using the bread to soak up the oil.

Per serving: Calories 225 (From Fat 86); Fat 10g (Saturated 2g); Cholesterol 239mg; Sodium 1,077mg; Carbohydrate 7g (Dietary Fiber 1g); Protein 27g.

CLEANING AND DEVEINING SHRIMP

Figure 9-1:
Cleaning and deveining shrimp.

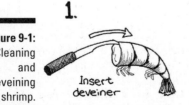

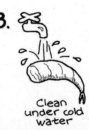

Illustration by Elizabeth Kurtzman

Bean Stuffed Chia Peppers

Prep time: 15 min • **Cook time:** 30 min • **Yield:** 6 servings

Ingredients	Directions
6 small red or yellow bell peppers	**1** Blanch the whole peppers in boiling water for 2 to 3 minutes to soften them a little. Carefully cut around the stalks of the peppers to make lids, making sure to keep the peppers intact and remove all the seeds.
2 tablespoons olive oil	
1 medium onion, chopped	**2** Preheat the oven to 350 degrees.
2 cloves garlic, finely sliced	**3** In a large frying pan, heat 1 tablespoon of the oil over medium heat; add the onion to the pan and cook for 5 minutes, until soft. Add the garlic and cook for another 2 or 3 minutes.
6 large ripe tomatoes	
One 15-ounce can pinto beans, drained and rinsed	
¼ cup chopped cilantro	**4** Meanwhile, score an X on the bottom of each tomato, place them in a large bowl, and pour boiling water over them; leave for approximately 4 to 5 minutes, until the skins come away easily. Remove the skins from the tomatoes and chop the flesh roughly. Add the tomatoes to the frying pan and simmer for 1 or 2 minutes. Remove the pan from the heat.
1 teaspoon ground cumin	
1 teaspoon hot smoked paprika	
2 tablespoons whole chia seeds	
Salt and pepper, to taste	
	5 Add the beans to the pan and roughly mash a few of them with a fork, leaving most of them whole. Add the chopped cilantro, cumin, paprika, chia, salt, and pepper and stir well. Stuff this mixture into the peppers and replace their lids.
	6 Oil a baking sheet with the remaining 1 tablespoon of oil. Lay the stuffed peppers on the baking sheet and cook in the oven for 20 minutes. Serve hot from the oven.

Per serving: Calories 190 (From Fat 61); Fat 7g (Saturated 1g); Cholesterol 0mg; Sodium 226mg; Carbohydrate 27g (Dietary Fiber 9g); Protein 7g.

Smoked Salmon and Dill Chia Tartlets

Prep time: 40 min • **Cook time:** 20 min • **Yield:** 6 servings

Ingredients	Directions
Butter, for greasing the trays	*1* Grease six 3½-inch loose-bottomed fluted tart tins with butter.
1½ cups flour	
Pinch of salt	*2* In a food processor, combine the flour, a pinch of salt, and the cold butter and process until the mixture resembles fine breadcrumbs. Transfer the mixture to a bowl and add enough very cold water to bring the dough together. Tip the dough onto a floured surface and divide into 6 equal parts. Roll out each piece of dough to fit the tart tins, and carefully put each pastry into the tart tins, pressing into the edges to fit the tin. Remove any excess dough, and put the rolling pin over each tin.
⅓ cup cold butter	
Very cold water	
½ cup sour cream	
1 teaspoon English mustard	
1 teaspoon lemon juice	
2 teaspoons capers, chopped	
3 egg yolks, lightly beaten	*3* Cut 6 disks of baking paper to fit each of the tins, put them over the pastry, and fill with dried beans to weigh down the paper. Chill in the refrigerator for at least 30 minutes.
⅔ cup smoked salmon, chopped roughly	
2 tablespoons whole chia seeds	*4* Preheat the oven to 400 degrees.
1 bunch fresh dill, chopped finely	*5* Bake the tart case blind in the oven for 10 minutes, and then remove the beans and baking paper.
Salt and pepper, to taste	*6* Meanwhile, in a large bowl, combine the sour cream, mustard, lemon juice, capers, egg yolks, smoked salmon, chia, dill, salt, and pepper; mix well.
	7 Divide the mixture evenly among the 6 tart cases, and return to the oven for 15 minutes more. Remove from the oven and cool in the tins for 5 minutes before serving.

Per serving: Calories 305 (From Fat 162); Fat 18g (Saturated 10g); Cholesterol 132mg; Sodium 391mg; Carbohydrate 27g (Dietary Fiber 2g); Protein 9g.

Carrot, Cabbage, and Chia Spring Rolls

Prep time: 15 min • **Cook time:** 20 min • **Yield:** 8 servings

Ingredients	Directions
2 large carrots	*1* Peel the carrots, and grate them using a wide grater blade.
1 tablespoon olive oil	
1 large onion, chopped	*2* In a large frying pan, heat the olive oil over medium heat, and cook the onion and garlic for 1 minute. Add the mustard seeds, chilies, fennel seeds, cumin seeds, cinnamon, and nutmeg, and cook for another 1 minute. Add the carrot, cabbage, and orange rind, and cook for another 1 minute. Remove from the heat, add the chia, and season with salt.
4 cloves garlic, thinly sliced	
2 teaspoons mustard seeds	
4 bird's eye chilies	
1 teaspoon fennel seeds	
1 tablespoon cumin seeds	
Pinch of cinnamon	*3* Lay a spring roll sheet on a clean work surface with a corner toward you, like a diamond shape. Spread a heaping tablespoon of the filling around 1½ inches from the bottom in a horizontal line around 4¾ inches long.
Pinch of nutmeg	
1 cup angel hair shredded cabbage	
Rind of 1 orange	*4* Fold the bottom half of the pastry over the filling and roll the pastry up tightly to just past the widest point of the pastry. Fold in the sides and brush with water before finishing the roll to the end.
2 tablespoons whole chia seeds	
Salt, to taste	*5* Repeat this process with the remaining pastry sheets.
8 spring roll pastry sheets	
Oil, for frying	*6* In a large frying pan, heat ¾ inch oil to around 350 degrees. Fry the spring rolls in the oil, turning once, until the pastry is crisp and lightly browned. You may need to repeat this a few times, depending on the size of the spring rolls and how they fit in the frying pan. Serve immediately.

Per serving: Calories 278 (From Fat 151); Fat 17g (Saturated 2g); Cholesterol 0mg; Sodium 276mg; Carbohydrate 27g (Dietary Fiber 4g); Protein 5g.

Avocado Bruschetta with Chia

Prep time: 10 min • **Cook time:** 30 min • **Yield:** 6 servings

Ingredients	*Directions*
½ cup balsamic vinegar	*1* Preheat the oven to 350 degrees.
1 tablespoon brown sugar	
1 baguette, sliced	*2* In a small saucepan, heat the balsamic vinegar and brown sugar over medium heat. Bring to a slight boil and simmer for 6 to 8 minutes, reducing the volume by half.
4 tablespoons olive oil	
1 clove garlic, halved lengthways	*3* On a large baking sheet, lay the bread and drizzle with 2 tablespoons of the olive oil. Bake until nearly toasted, for about 5 minutes; then rub all the slices with the garlic.
1 cup cherry tomatoes	
1 avocado	*4* Cut the cherry tomatoes into quarters and put them in a large bowl.
½ small red onion	
1 tablespoon whole chia seeds	*5* Cut the avocado in half, remove the stone, peel it, and cut it into ½-inch cubes. Add the avocado to the tomatoes.
1 teaspoon soft brown sugar	
Salt and pepper, to taste	*6* Thinly slice the red onion and add to the bowl.
1 handful fresh basil leaves	
	7 Add the remaining 2 tablespoons of olive oil to the bowl, along with the chia and brown sugar; mix well. Season with salt and pepper to taste, and divide the mixture between the bread slices.
	8 Wash and roughly tear the basil leaves.
	9 Serve the bruschetta along with the torn basil leaves and drizzle over the balsamic reduction over the finished bruschetta.

Per serving: Calories 348 (From Fat 119); Fat 13g (Saturated 2g); Cholesterol 0mg; Sodium 530mg; Carbohydrate 50g (Dietary Fiber 4g); Protein 10g.

Soups

Soups and chia seeds have two things in common:

- ✔ They're ancient foods.
- ✔ They're nutritionally dense.

The idea of putting a mix of meats, vegetables, beans, fish, and many other foods into a pot, flavoring it, and serving up to your family is an ancient tradition. All over the world, different cultures are famous for their varieties in soups. The Italians are famous for their pasta soups, Americans are known for their chowders, bean soups are cooked all over South America and Central America, and the Asian countries certainly know how to mix their delicate flavors and spices into wonderful soups. These soup recipes are passed down through the generations, often changed along the way, but always remaining a great source of nutrition.

By simply mixing fresh produce with various herbs and spices and adding chia seeds, you can make fabulous-tasting soups filled with the nutrients your body needs to function well and keep you feeling revitalized and energetic. The versatility of soups mean that you can literally use whatever vegetables you have left over in your cupboard. An onion, garlic, some celery, carrots, and potato make a wonderful soup if mixed with a good vegetable stock, some herbs, and chia seeds. It's that simple. You can then take your soup to work, pack it in your kid's thermos for school, or pop it in the freezer to use at your convenience. There really are no excuses for not eating good food when it comes to soups — they're simple, nutritious bowls of goodness that can be served as appetizers or made as heartier main meals.

Butter Bean and Leek Soup

Prep time: 10 min • **Cook time:** 30 min • **Yield:** 6 servings

Ingredients	Directions
4 medium leeks	*1* Trim the leeks so that only the white and pale green part is left. Halve them lengthways and slice thinly. Wash the leeks thoroughly, separating the rings.
1 tablespoon olive oil	
1 tablespoon butter	
2 teaspoons chopped fresh thyme	*2* In a large saucepan, heat the olive oil and butter over medium heat; add the leeks.
1 bay leaf	*3* Add the thyme and bay leaf to the saucepan. Cook for about 10 minutes, until soft.
3 garlic cloves, finely chopped	
½ red chili, seeds removed and finely chopped	*4* Add the garlic and chili to the saucepan and cook for another 2 minutes.
5 cups vegetable stock	*5* Add the vegetable stock to the saucepan.
Two 15-ounce cans butter beans, drained	*6* Drain and rinse the butter beans; add them to the saucepan.
2 teaspoons oregano	*7* Wash and roughly chop the oregano and parsley; add them to the saucepan.
3 tablespoons parsley	
Salt and pepper, to taste	*8* Add the salt and pepper and bring the soup to a simmer, cooking for another 20 minutes.
3 tablespoons whole chia seeds	*9* Remove the bay leaf and adjust the seasoning to taste.
	10 Serve in deep bowls and top each serving with ½ tablespoon whole chia seeds.

Per serving: Calories 167 (From Fat 54); Fat 6g (Saturated 2g); Cholesterol 5mg; Sodium 1,190mg; Carbohydrate 28g (Dietary Fiber 7g); Protein 5g.

Soup of Curried Parsnip and Green Vegetables

Prep time: 10 min • **Cook time:** 30 min • **Yield:** 6 servings

Ingredients	Directions
2 tablespoons olive oil	**1** In a large saucepan, heat the olive oil over medium heat.
1 large onion	
2 tablespoons butter	**2** Peel and finely chop the onion; add it to the saucepan and cook for approximately 10 minutes, until soft. Turn down the heat, add the butter, and heat until melted.
2 tablespoons curry powder	
2 tablespoons milled chia seeds	
5 cups vegetable stock	**3** Remove the saucepan from the heat and add the curry powder and chia; stir well. Pour in the vegetable stock and return to medium heat to bring to a boil.
3 medium parsnips	
½ cup sour cream	**4** Peel and dice the parsnips into approximately 1-inch cubes; add them to the saucepan, and simmer for 20 minutes.
½ cup green beans	
½ cup peas, fresh or frozen	
1 handful baby spinach leaves	**5** Remove the saucepan from the heat and blend everything using a hand blender.
	6 Stir in the sour cream and heat to a near simmer.
	7 Trim the green beans, and cut into 1-inch fingers. Add the green beans and peas to the soup and cook for another 6 minutes.
	8 Add the spinach and stir well; cook for another 1 minute until the spinach wilts.

Per serving: Calories 211 (From Fat 113); Fat 13g (Saturated 5g); Cholesterol 19mg; Sodium 1,012mg; Carbohydrate 24g (Dietary Fiber 6g); Protein 3g.

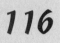

Tomato and Lentil Soup

Prep time: 10 min • **Cook time:** 30 min • **Yield:** 6 servings

Ingredients	Directions
2 tablespoons olive oil	*1* In a large saucepan, heat the olive oil over medium heat.
2 carrots, peeled and roughly chopped	
2 sticks celery, sliced	*2* Add the carrots, celery, and onion to the pan. Cook for about 10 minutes, until the onion is soft.
1 large onion, peeled and roughly chopped	
3 cloves garlic, finely chopped	*3* Add the garlic to the saucepan; cook for another 1 minute.
5 cups vegetable stock	*4* Add the vegetable stock to the saucepan, and bring to a boil.
¾ cup red lentils	
Two 15-ounce cans plum tomatoes	*5* Add the lentils, canned tomatoes, and whole tomatoes. Return to a boil and simmer for 15 minutes, stirring occasionally.
6 large ripe tomatoes, stems removed and roughly chopped	
1 small bunch fresh basil	*6* Remove the soup from the heat and add the basil and chia.
2 tablespoons milled chia seeds	*7* Add the salt and pepper.
Salt and pepper, to taste	*8* Using a hand blender, blend everything until smooth.

Per serving: Calories 236 (From Fat 53); Fat 6g (Saturated 1g); Cholesterol 0mg; Sodium 1,155mg; Carbohydrate 36g (Dietary Fiber 10g); Protein 10g.

Note: If you think the consistency of the soup is too thick, add more water or vegetable stock and return to a boil for 1 minute before serving.

Tip: Spoon some sour cream over each serving to add color and creamy goodness.

Salads

Salads are where it's at when it comes to healthy eating. By eating plenty of different types of fruits and vegetables, you're guaranteeing that your body is getting plenty of the good stuff like fiber, vitamins, and minerals. That's why trying to get your whole family to love salads is so important — you want salads to be an integral part of their diets and yours! By choosing fresh produce, mixing up different flavors and textures, and making sure that you use a tasty dressing, you're well on your way to enticing even the pickiest eaters in your house. Although salads are often served before a main meal or as a side dish, there's no reason you can't make them the main course — just beef them up with different meats, cheeses, nuts, seeds, olives, and many more delicious foods.

The basics to a good salad are fresh produce and a good mix of flavor and textures, but chia seeds are always a welcome addition. We like to use whole chia seeds in salads because the seeds add a little crunch and pack in the nutrients without affecting the flavor. However, if you prefer milled chia seeds, simply mix the milled seeds with the salad dressing before dressing the salad, and you can still benefit from all the extra nutrients.

The recipes in this section are a small sample of what you can do with a salad to mix up different cooked and raw vegetables. Salad combinations are limitless, so whatever salads you and your family enjoy, start welcoming chia seeds into the mix and reaping their health benefits!

Chia Chicken and Avocado Salad with Honey Mustard Dressing

Prep time: 15 min • **Yield:** 2 servings

Ingredients	Directions
2 boneless, skinless chicken breasts	**1** Slice the chicken breasts into thin, long strips and season well with salt and pepper. In a frying pan, heat the oil over medium heat; add the chicken strips to the pan and cook for 8 to 10 minutes, stirring occasionally until the chicken is nicely browned and cooked through. Set aside.
Salt and pepper, to taste	
2 tablespoons olive oil	
2 cups chopped spinach	**2** In a large bowl, combine the spinach and baby salad leaves.
2 cups mixed baby salad leaves	
1 cup cherry tomatoes	**3** Wash and cut the cherry tomatoes in half. Peel the avocado and cut it into slices, removing and discarding the center stone. Add the tomatoes, avocado, cheese, pine nuts, and chia to the bowl of salad leaves.
1 large avocado	
½ cup crumbled feta cheese	
¼ cup toasted pine nuts	
2 tablespoons whole chia seeds	**4** Pour the Honey Mustard Dressing over the salad and mix everything together with clean hands so that all the leaves get dressed with the oil. Add the cooked chicken strips on top. Serve immediately.
Honey Mustard Dressing (see the following recipe)	

Honey Mustard Dressing

2 tablespoons extra-virgin olive oil	**1** In a small mason jar, mix all the ingredients.
1 tablespoon freshly squeezed lemon juice	**2** Put the lid on the jar, and shake vigorously until well combined.
1 teaspoon English mustard	
1 teaspoon honey	
Salt and pepper, to taste	

Per serving: Calories 878 (From Fat 610); Fat 68g (Saturated 14g); Cholesterol 107mg; Sodium 765mg; Carbohydrate 32g (Dietary Fiber 16g); Protein 42g.

Roasted Root Vegetable Salad with Balsamic Dressing

Prep time: 15 min • **Cook time:** 40 min • **Yield:** 4 servings

Ingredients	Directions
1 medium sweet potato	*1* Preheat the oven to 350 degrees.
½ butternut squash	
1 red bell pepper	*2* Peel the skin from the sweet potato and chop into 1-inch cubes. Peel the butternut squash, discard the seeds, and chop into 1-inch cubes. Wash the bell pepper, remove the stalk and seeds, and cut into large strips.
3 tablespoons olive oil	
1 small bunch rosemary, finely chopped	
1 small bunch thyme, finely chopped	*3* In a large roasting dish, combine the sweet potato, butternut squash, and bell peppers and pour over the olive oil, stirring well so everything gets coated with oil. Sprinkle over the rosemary, thyme, salt, and pepper. Roast for approximately 40 minutes, until cooked through.
Salt and pepper, to taste	
6 cups salad leaves	
½ red onion, thinly sliced	
Balsamic Dressing (see the following recipe)	*4* In a large bowl, add the salad leaves and onion, cover with half the Balsamic Dressing, and mix well. When the vegetables are cooked nicely, divide the dressed salad between 4 plates and top each plate evenly with the roasted vegetables. Sprinkle the chia seeds evenly among each salad to serve.
2 tablespoons whole chia seeds	

Balsamic Dressing

6 tablespoons extra-virgin olive oil	*1* In a mason jar, mix all the ingredients.
2 tablespoons balsamic vinegar	*2* Put the lid on the jar, and shake vigorously until well combined.
1 garlic clove, peeled and minced	
1 teaspoon dark brown sugar	

Per serving: Calories 302 (From Fat 196); Fat 22g (Saturated 3g); Cholesterol 0mg; Sodium 360mg; Carbohydrate 24g (Dietary Fiber 6g); Protein 4g.

Spicy Chorizo and Goat Cheese Chia Salad with Herb Dressing

Prep time: 20 min • **Cook time:** 10 min • **Yield:** 4 servings

Ingredients	Directions
1 cup goat cheese	*1* On an ovenproof plate, place the goat cheese and top with pepper. Place the plate under a medium grill for about 8 minutes, until the cheese is melted.
Pepper, to taste	
1 tablespoon olive oil	
One whole 8-ounce chorizo sausage	*2* In a frying pan, heat the oil over medium heat; add the sausage and fry for about 5 minutes, until the juices start to run. Remove the sausage from the pan and slice it thinly and again in half so they're semicircle-shaped small pieces. Set aside.
1 cup cherry tomatoes	
½ cup pickled beetroot, drained	
6 cups baby salad leaves	*3* Cut the cherry tomatoes in half and add to the frying pan that the sausage was cooked in; cook for 1 minute so that the juices from the sausage cover the tomatoes and they start to cook. Remove the tomatoes from the heat and set aside.
¼ cup hazelnuts, lightly toasted	
2 tablespoons whole chia seeds	
Herb Dressing (see the following recipe)	*4* Chop the beetroot into 1-inch cubes and place on paper towel to absorb the excess liquid. Put the salad leaves on a large serving plate, and top with the beetroot, hazelnuts, and chia. Sprinkle the sausage and tomatoes over the salad. Scatter the goat cheese on top of the salad. Pour the Herb Dressing over the salad. Serve immediately.

Herb Dressing

6 tablespoons extra-virgin olive oil	*1* In a mason jar, combine all the ingredients.
2 tablespoons red wine vinegar	*2* Put the lid on the jar and shake vigorously until well combined.
1 tablespoon chopped parsley	
1 teaspoon honey	
Salt and pepper, to taste	

Per serving: Calories 672 (From Fat 529); Fat 59g (Saturated 17g); Cholesterol 85mg; Sodium 1,059mg; Carbohydrate 13g (Dietary Fiber 5g); Protein 22g.

Drinks

You may think you're eating a healthy diet if you load up on fresh fruits and vegetables, keep saturated fats to a minimum, and get healthy fats, but watching what you're drinking is important, too. It's easy to drink way too many calories without even realizing it. No matter how healthy your food intake is, if you're drinking sugary sodas all day, you're putting your health at risk.

 Avoid sugary drinks that have no nutrient value whatsoever. Instead, try to make water your main drink. Drink it hot with some freshly squeezed lemon juice in the mornings instead of your usual tea or coffee.

If you're entertaining or you need a sweet treat, add chia seeds to your drinks. That way, you can be sure you're adding to your nutritional requirements for the day.

Classic Chia Fresca

Prep time: 5 min • **Yield:** 1 serving

Ingredients	Directions
1 lime	**1** Roll the lime along the countertop before cutting; then cut the lime in half and squeeze out the juice. The rolling helps soften the fruit and helps you get more juice.
1 tablespoon sugar	
1 cup water	
1 tablespoon whole chia seeds	**2** Pour the lime juice into a tall glass and add the sugar.
Ice, to serve	**3** Add the water and stir well, until the sugar dissolves.
	4 Add the chia and stir again.
	5 Serve with ice immediately or, if you prefer, you can leave the chia seeds to become gelatinous for about 15 minutes before serving.

Per serving: Calories 108 (From Fat 29); Fat 3g (Saturated 0g); Cholesterol 0mg; Sodium 2mg; Carbohydrate 20g (Dietary Fiber 5g); Protein 2g.

Vary It! This is a recipe for classic chia fresca, but for a healthier version, simply swap the sugar for a substitute of your choice, such as stevia.

Tip: For a more nutritious drink, try using coconut water instead of plain water.

Chia fresca: The original energy drink

Chia fresca has been around for centuries. It's made by mixing lime or lemon juice with chia seeds, water, and some sort of sweetener. The Tarahumara Indians of Mexico's Copper Canyon are famous for this classic drink. They use it to help fuel their epic runs — sometimes over 100 miles in a day. Today, chia fresca is served in many towns right across Central America and South America as a refreshing drink, but it's also well known for it's energy-giving benefits. As chia's popularity grows across western countries, chia fresca is fast becoming the natural but healthy substitute to commercial energy drinks.

Strawberry Lemonade

Prep time: 20 min • **Yield:** 8 servings

Ingredients	Directions
1½ cups sugar	**1** In a medium saucepan, mix the sugar with the lemon zest and 1 cup of the water. Heat over medium heat and simmer for 5 minutes, stirring occasionally.
Zest of 2 lemons	
5 cups cold water	**2** Remove from the heat and allow to cool completely. Set aside.
1 cup fresh strawberries	
2 cups freshly squeezed lemon juice (approximately 8 lemons)	**3** Meanwhile, wash the strawberries and remove the green hull.
3 tablespoons whole chia seeds	**4** Place the strawberries and 1 cup of the cold water in a blender and blend on high for a few seconds.
2 cups ice, to serve	**5** Add the strawberry mixture to the freshly squeezed lemon juice.
	6 Add the cooled simple syrup to the lemon juice and strawberry mixture.
	7 Add the remaining 3 cups of water and the chia; stir well.
	8 Serve in a large pitcher with ice.

Per serving: Calories 187 (From Fat 13); Fat 1g (Saturated 0g); Cholesterol 0mg; Sodium 2mg; Carbohydrate 46g (Dietary Fiber 2g); Protein 1g.

Tip: Serve this pitcher of lemonade within an hour of making it. The chia seeds will begin to turn gelatinous, and you're better off enjoying the drink before it gets too thick.

Vary It! Although the recipe uses plain water, it's also delicious when made with sparkling water, such as San Pellegrino. So, if you love the bubbles, use sparkling water instead.

Pick-Me-Up Party Punch

Prep time: 20 min • **Yield:** 16 servings

Ingredients	Directions
¹⁄₃ cup whole chia seeds	**1** In a small bowl, mix the chia and the water and stir well. Leave this mixture to thicken for 15 minutes, stirring occasionally until it forms a chia gel.
2 cups water	
2 cups peach schnapps, chilled	**2** In a large bowl, combine the peach schnapps, vodka, pineapple juice, orange juice, and cranberry juice; stir.
4 cups vodka, chilled	
2 cups pineapple juice, chilled	**3** Add the orange bitters to the large bowl, if desired.
4 cups orange juice, chilled	
1 cup cranberry juice, chilled	**4** Roll the limes along a countertop to soften the fruit. Slice 2 of the limes in half and squeeze out the juice. Add this lime juice to the large bowl.
1 tablespoon orange bitters (optional)	
4 limes	**5** Add to the large bowl the chia gel that you made earlier and stir well so that the chia gel is mixed in evenly.
2 lemons	
3 oranges	**6** Slice the other 2 limes thinly and add to the large bowl.
1 cup strawberries	**7** Slice the lemons and oranges thinly and add to the bowl.
A small bunch of fresh mint leaves	
8 cups ice	**8** Remove the green hull from the strawberries and wash well. Cut the strawberries into quarters lengthways and add them to the large bowl.
	9 Wash the mint leaves and tear apart roughly before adding them to the large bowl.
	10 Mix everything together and add the ice before serving in a large punch bowl with a soup ladle.

Per serving: Calories 284 (From Fat 11); Fat 1g (Saturated 0g); Cholesterol 0mg; Sodium 5mg; Carbohydrate 20g (Dietary Fiber 3g); Protein 1g.

Nutty Banana Milkshake

Prep time: 10 min • **Yield:** 2 servings

Ingredients	Directions
2 bananas	**1** Slice the bananas and put most of them in a blender. Set aside some of the sliced bananas for garnish.
2 tablespoons chopped almonds	
2 cups milk	**2** To the blender, add the almonds, milk, ice cream, milled chia seeds, maple syrup, and cinnamon.
1 cup vanilla ice cream	
1 tablespoon milled chia seeds	**3** Blend on high for approximately 1 minute, until everything is well combined.
2 tablespoons pure maple syrup	
½ teaspoon cinnamon	**4** Add the ice and blend again until the mixture is thick.
½ cup ice	
Whole chia seeds, for garnish	**5** Divide the milkshake between 2 tall glasses and garnish with the sliced banana you saved from earlier and the whole chia seeds.
	6 Serve immediately with a long-handled teaspoon.

Per serving: *Calories 498 (From Fat 179); Fat 20g (Saturated 10g); Cholesterol 53mg; Sodium 162mg; Carbohydrate 71g (Dietary Fiber 6g); Protein 20g.*

Vary It! If you're not a fan of bananas, simply swap them for strawberries, peaches, or whatever other fruits are in season.

Chapter 10

Mouthwatering Main Courses and Sides

- -

In This Chapter

▶ Preparing tasty but simple one-pot dinners

▶ Making meat your main course

▶ Serving up the best of seafood

▶ Adding a little something on the side

- -

Whenever you enjoy your main meal — whether midday or late in the evening — it's probably the meal that you spend the most time preparing. You're trying to pack in as many healthy nutrients as possible without overloading on saturated fats or sugars. If you're the one who cooks most of the main meals in your household, this chapter will give you ideas on how to provide good, wholesome, tasty meals that don't take all day to prepare.

In this chapter, we give you recipes that are easy to make and packed full of healthy ingredients with a good mix of spice and flavor. By adding chia seeds to your main meals, you pack in extra nutrients that are essential to keep your family healthy and full of energy.

One-Pot Wonders

Sometimes all you really need is one pot to make a delicious meal. One-pot recipes are fantastic for making more of what you need and getting two or three days out of one recipe. Just refrigerate it and reheat it the next day — it'll probably taste even better because the ingredients have had a chance to mingle longer.

Braised Lamb Shanks with Cannellini Beans

Prep time: 15 min • **Cook time:** 2½ hr • **Yield:** 4 servings

Ingredients	Directions
2 tablespoons olive oil	*1* Preheat the oven to 325 degrees.
1 large onion, thinly sliced	
4 large lamb shanks	*2* In a large ovenproof casserole dish or Dutch oven, heat the oil and sauté the onion for 5 minutes.
4 carrots, peeled and chopped	
2 celery sticks, trimmed and thinly sliced	*3* Add the lamb shanks and cook for 5 minutes, until the lamb is browned on all sides. Remove the lamb shanks with a slotted spoon and set aside.
1 garlic clove, peeled and crushed	
One 15-ounce can cannellini beans, drained and rinsed	*4* Add the carrots and celery to the dish, and sauté the vegetables for another 5 minutes.
One 15-ounce can chopped tomatoes	*5* Add the garlic to the dish, and cook for another 1 minute.
1 cup red wine	*6* Return the lamb shanks to the dish. Add the beans, tomatoes, and wine to the dish and stir well.
Zest and juice of 1 orange	
2 bay leaves	*7* Add to the dish the orange zest and juice, bay leaves, rosemary, and vegetable stock and stir well. Bring to a boil, and then cover the dish and cook in the oven for 1 hour.
1 small bunch of rosemary	
1 cup vegetable stock	
2 tablespoons whole chia seeds	*8* Turn the lamb shanks over in the stock, and return to the oven for another 1½ hours, until the lamb is tender.
Salt and pepper, to taste	*9* Remove the bay leaf, add the chia, season with salt and pepper, and stir well to combine the seeds evenly throughout the dish.
2 tablespoons chopped parsley, for garnish	
	10 Garnish with parsley and serve hot from the oven.

Per serving: Calories 597 (From Fat 254); Fat 28g (Saturated 9g); Cholesterol 157mg; Sodium 916mg; Carbohydrate 34g (Dietary Fiber 11g); Protein 50g.

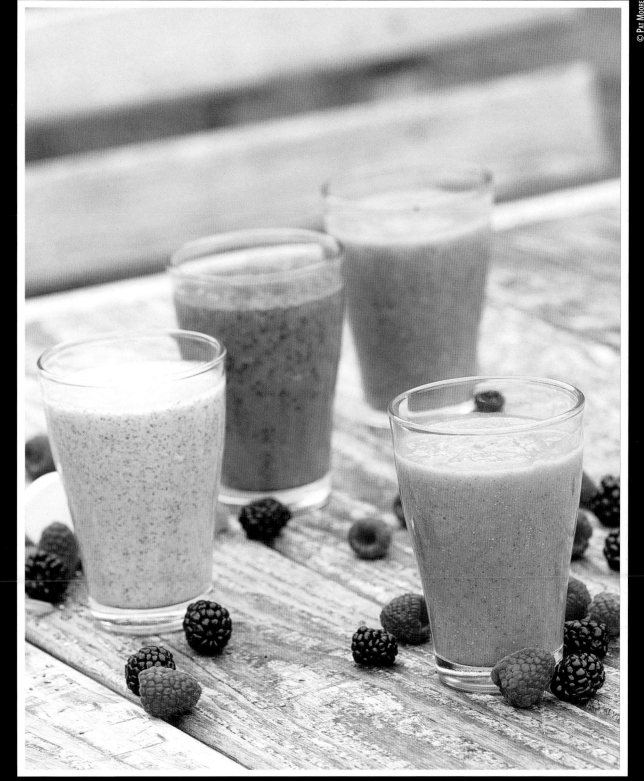

Standard Protein Smoothie, Coffee Smoothie, Green Fruit and Veggie Smoothie Combo, and Healthy Carrot Cardio Smoothie (all in Chapter 8)

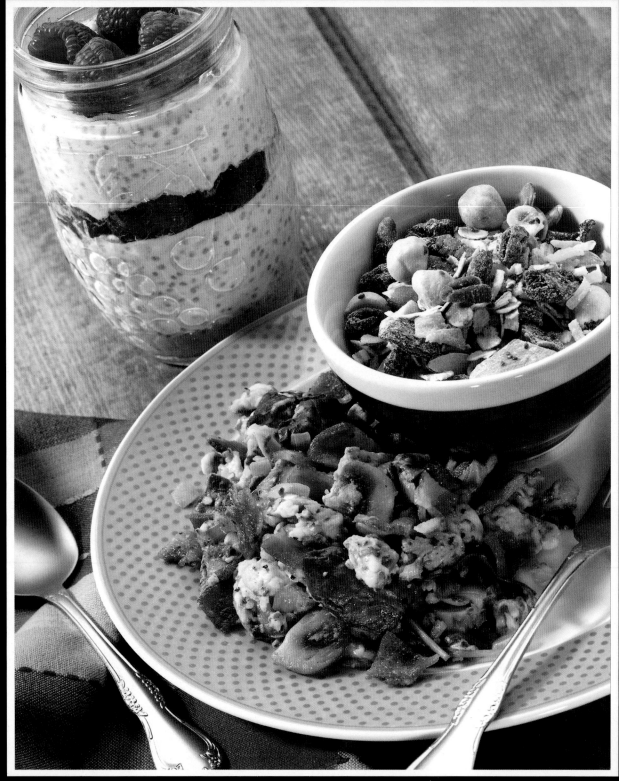

Overnight Oats (Chapter 6), Mega Muesli (Chapter 6), and Hearty Chia Breakfast Eggs (Chapter 7)

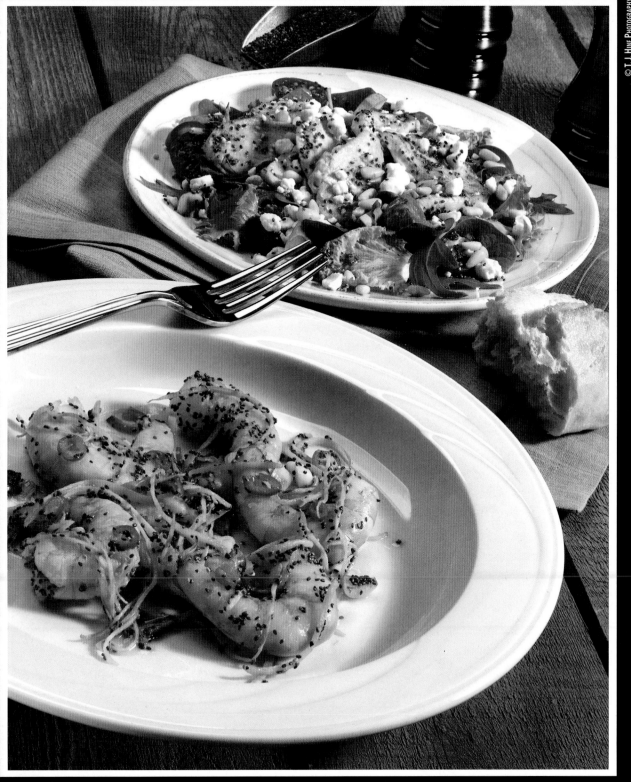

Chia Chicken and Avocado Salad with Honey Mustard Dressing and Spicy Ginger Prawns (both in Chapter 9)

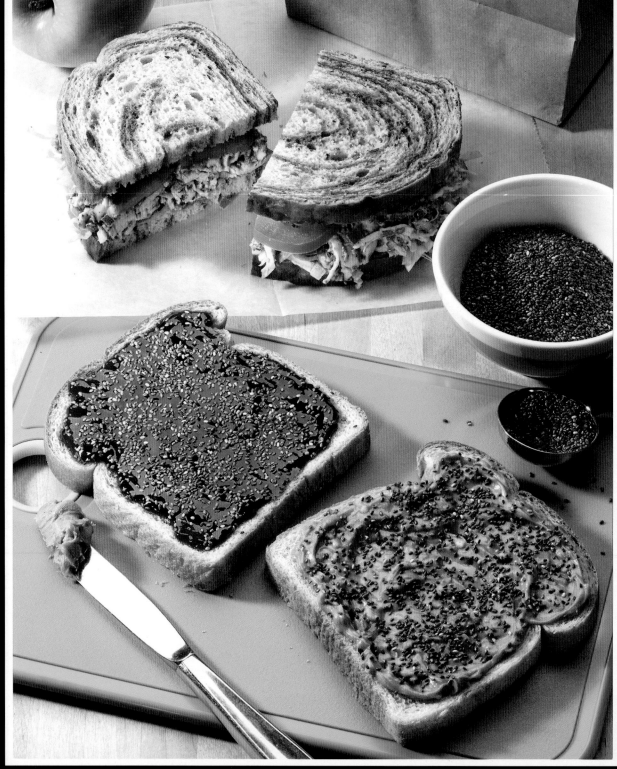

Pesto Chicken Sandwich and Classic Peanut Butter and Jelly Sandwich (both in Chapter 14)

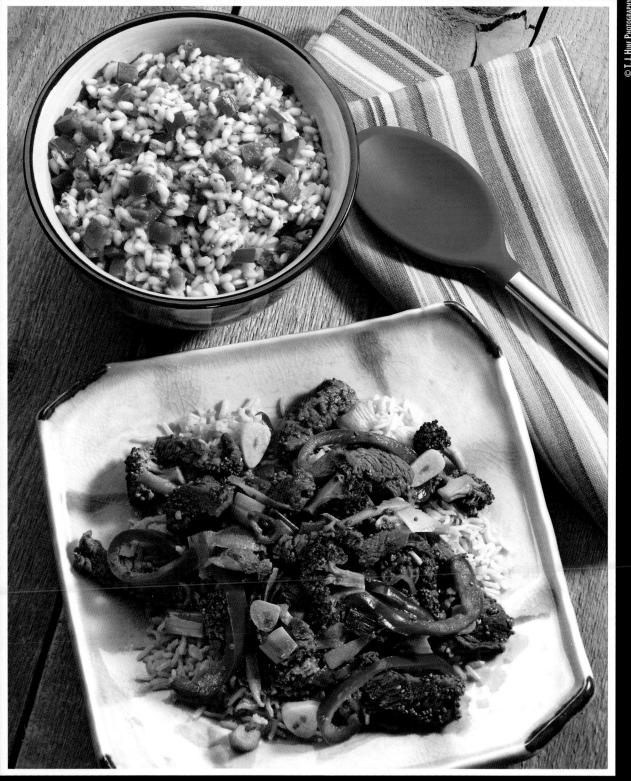

© T. J. Hine Photography

Red Pepper Risotto and Spicy Thai Beef (both in Chapter 10)

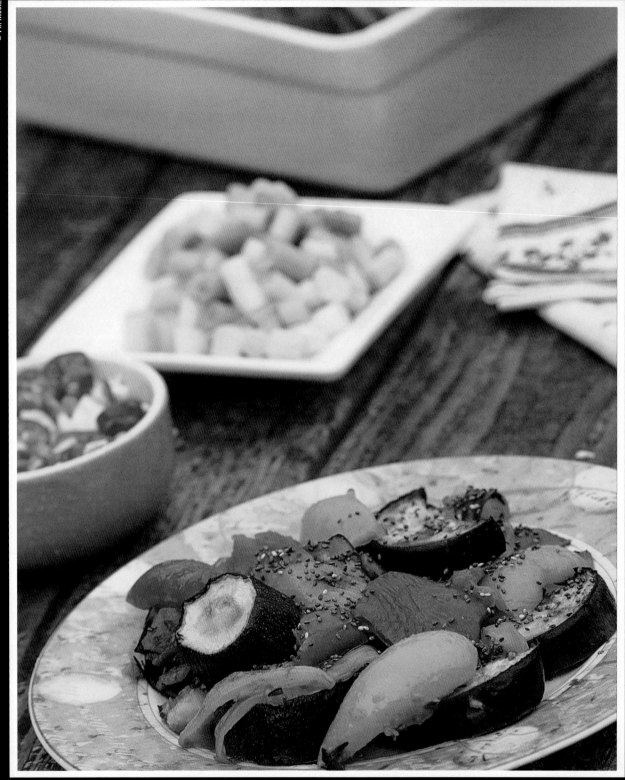

Chia Ratatouille (Chapter 10)

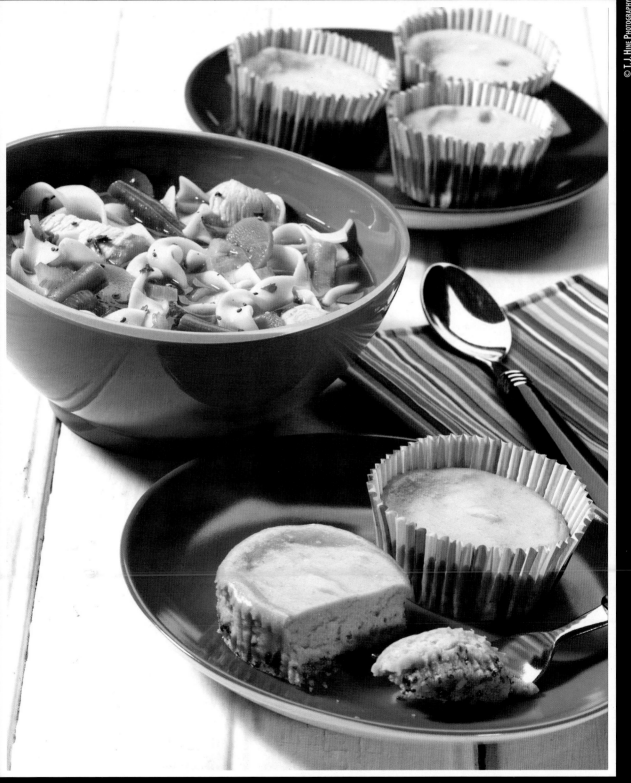

Chicken Noodle Soup and Mini Baked Raspberry Cheesecakes (both in Chapter 12)

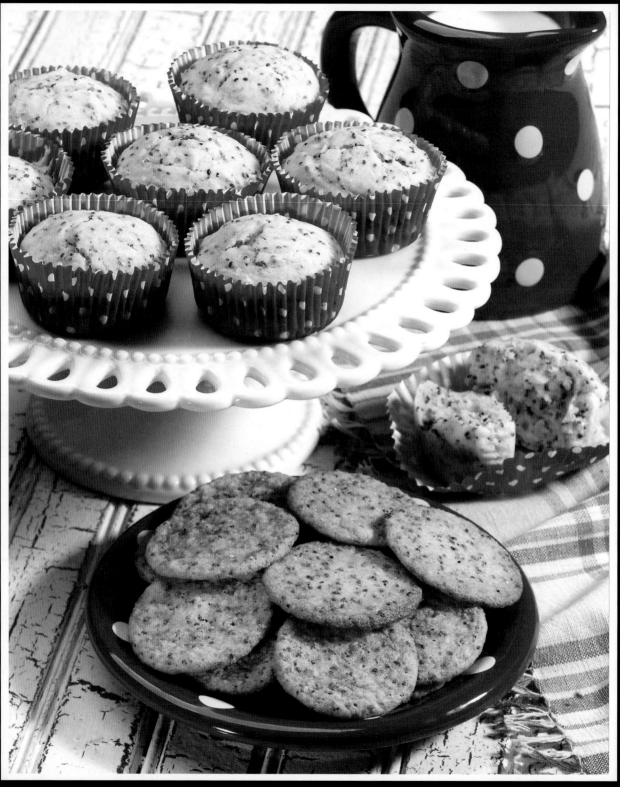

Lemon and Chia Cupcakes and Chia Cookies (both in Chapter 15)

Beef and Guinness Stew with Horseradish Dumplings

Prep time: 15 min • **Cook time:** 2½ hr • **Yield:** 8 servings

Ingredients	Directions
2 tablespoons olive oil	*1* Preheat the oven to 325 degrees.
2 pounds stewing beef in large chunks	*2* In a large ovenproof casserole dish or Dutch oven, heat the oil and brown the beef in batches until it's well browned. Remove the beef and set aside. Add the carrots and leeks to the dish and cook for 4 to 5 minutes. Add the barley, Guinness, and beef stock to the dish. Return the beef to the dish and season with salt and pepper. Bring to a boil, cover, and cook in the oven for 2 hours. Check occasionally, adding more beef stock if necessary.
4 carrots, peeled and sliced	
2 large leeks, sliced	
¼ cup pearl barley	
1½ cups Guinness or other stout	
3 cups beef stock	
Salt and pepper, to taste	*3* In a large frying pan, sauté the onion in the butter for 10 minutes, until soft. Transfer the sautéed onions to a bowl and add the finely chopped parsley, breadcrumbs, egg, and horseradish. Using clean hands, bring the mixture together and form 12 small dumpling balls.
½ onion, finely chopped	
1 tablespoon butter	
4 tablespoons finely chopped parsley	
1 cup breadcrumbs	*4* Remove the dish from the oven, add the chia, and stir well. Dot the dumplings on top of the beef, cover, and return to the oven for 20 minutes. Remove the lid of the casserole and return to the oven for another 10 minutes. Garnish with parsley and serve hot from the oven.
1 large egg	
3 tablespoons creamed horseradish	
2 tablespoons whole chia seeds	
2 tablespoon chopped parsley, to garnish	

Per serving: Calories 308 (From Fat 111); Fat 12g (Saturated 4g); Cholesterol 82mg; Sodium 659mg; Carbohydrate 25g (Dietary Fiber 4g); Protein 25g.

Creamy Chia Chicken

Prep time: 15 min • **Cook time:** 1 hr 25 min • **Yield:** 8 servings

Ingredients	Directions
½ cup diced bacon pieces, uncooked	*1* Preheat the oven to 325 degrees.
8 pieces of chicken on the bone (breasts, thighs, drumsticks)	*2* In a large ovenproof casserole dish or Dutch oven over high heat, add the bacon pieces. Cook for about 1 minute, until the fat starts to come out of the bacon.
2 tablespoon milled chia seeds	
½ cup dry white wine	*3* Add the chicken pieces and cook for 5 to 10 minutes, turning occasionally until lightly browned.
1 cup vegetable stock	
2 large leeks	*4* Sprinkle the chia over the chicken and stir well.
1 pound new potatoes	*5* Add the wine and scrape the bottom of the dish to incorporate all the juices from the cooking.
6 tablespoons sour cream	
2 teaspoon Dijon mustard	*6* Add the vegetable stock and bring to a boil.
2 tablespoons chopped fresh tarragon	*7* Wash and trim the leeks and cut into 1-inch pieces.
Salt and pepper, to taste	*8* Wash the potatoes and add to the dish with the leeks.
	9 Add the sour cream and Dijon mustard to the dish and return to a simmer.
	10 Cover the dish, lower the heat, and gently simmer for another 15 minutes.
	11 Place the dish in the oven for 1 hour.
	12 Remove the dish from the oven, add the tarragon; and stir well. Season with salt and pepper.

Per serving: *Calories 242 (From Fat 60); Fat 7g (Saturated 2g); Cholesterol 81mg; Sodium 349mg; Carbohydrate 14g (Dietary Fiber 2g); Protein 30g.*

Tip: Serve freshly steamed greens such as broccoli or snap peas on the side of this dish to add more nutrients.

Chia and Chickpea Hotpot

Prep time: 10 min • **Cook time:** 50 min • **Yield:** 6 servings

Ingredients	*Directions*
3 tablespoons olive oil	*1* Preheat the oven to 325 degrees.
1 large onion, chopped	
1 large turnip, peeled and trimmed	*2* In a large ovenproof casserole dish or Dutch oven, heat the oil over medium heat; add the onion to cook for 10 minutes until soft.
½ butternut squash	
2 garlic cloves, peeled and crushed	*3* Chop the turnip into 1-inch cubes.
2 leeks, trimmed and sliced	*4* Peel the butternut squash, remove the core with all the seeds, and chop the flesh into 1-inch pieces.
3 carrots, trimmed and sliced	
2 sticks celery, trimmed and sliced	*5* Add the turnip, butternut squash, garlic, leeks, carrots, and celery to the dish and cook for another 5 minutes.
½ cup bulgur wheat	
One 15-ounce can chickpeas, drained and rinsed	*6* Stir in the bulgur, chickpeas, tomatoes, and chives. Add the vegetable stock and bring to a boil.
One 15-ounce can chopped tomatoes	
2 tablespoons chopped chives, plus extra for garnish	*7* Remove from the heat, cover, and place in the oven for 40 minutes.
2½ cups vegetable stock	*8* Remove the dish from the oven, add the chia seeds, and stir well.
2 tablespoons whole chia seeds	
	9 Garnish with chives.

Per serving: Calories 294 (From Fat 84); Fat 9g (Saturated 1g); Cholesterol 0mg; Sodium 691mg; Carbohydrate 49g (Dietary Fiber 9g); Protein 8g.

Note: We call for canned chickpeas in this recipe for ease of use, but if you prefer you can use dried chickpeas. Just soak them overnight in water and cook them according to the package instructions.

Red Pepper Risotto

Prep time: 10 min • **Cook time:** 25 min • **Yield:** 4 servings

Ingredients	Directions
1 tablespoon butter	*1* In a large saucepan over medium heat, melt the butter and olive oil.
1 tablespoon olive oil	
1 large onion, finely diced	*2* Add the onion and cook for 8 minutes; add the garlic and cook for another 2 minutes.
2 cloves garlic, peeled and crushed	
1 cup Arborio rice	*3* Add the rice and make sure it all gets coated in the butter.
½ cup dry white wine	
1 red bell pepper, stalks and seeds removed, finely diced	*4* Add the wine and cook while stirring for 1 minute, until the wine has evaporated.
4 cups chicken stock	*5* Add the bell pepper and cook for another 2 minutes.
Salt and pepper, to taste	
2 tablespoons whole chia seeds	*6* In a separate saucepan, warm the chicken stock over medium heat until it nearly reaches a simmer. Add 1 ladle of the chicken stock to the rice mixture and cook while stirring until it reduces down; add another ladle of the chicken stock to the rice mixture. Repeat, adding stock until it has absorbed, and then adding more when necessary. Continue stirring all the time while the rice is absorbing the stock.
Pinch of chili flakes	
¼ cup grated Parmesan cheese	
	7 Continue until the stock is gone and the rice is soft, tender, and creamy but still firm in the center. Season with salt and pepper.
	8 Remove from the heat, add the chia, and stir well. Stir in the chili flakes and cheese and serve.

Per serving: Calories 318 (From Fat 98); Fat 11g (Saturated 3g); Cholesterol 12mg; Sodium 1,156mg; Carbohydrate 47g (Dietary Fiber 5g); Protein 9g.

Meaty Mains

Humans have been eating meat since they learned how to. Meat is a great source of protein, the building block of life that we need to build muscle and regenerate every cell in our bodies. Often, meat takes center stage at meals, so it's important to choose your meats wisely.

Get to know your local butcher and make sure that any meat you purchase can be traced back to the farm it was produced from. That way you can be sure that you're getting what you ordered.

Here are some more tips for choosing meat:

- Avoid processed meats that have ingredients added that you don't recognize.
- Choose meats that don't have a lot of salt added.
- Don't eat fatty red meat every day; instead, choose leaner cuts and mix it up a bit with chicken or fish.

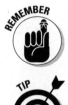

A varied diet is key to health so eating different meats can be part of a healthy diet, especially if you load up on vegetables along with your meat and add chia into the mix. That way, you'll be providing your body with a lot of the key nutrients it needs for good health.

In this section, we give you a mix of recipes for using beef, chicken, lamb, and pork. Most of the recipes have a bit of spice — if you're not fond of the heat, leave out the chilies.

Spicy Thai Beef

Prep time: 15 min • **Cook time:** 10 min • **Yield:** 4 servings

Ingredients	Directions
2 red chilies, thinly sliced	*1* In a large bowl, mix the chilies, soy sauce, fish sauce, and garlic.
¼ cup light soy sauce	
1½ tablespoons fish sauce	*2* Peel the ginger, cut it into matchstick-size pieces, and add it to the bowl. Add plenty of pepper.
6 cloves garlic, peeled and sliced	
One 2-inch piece fresh ginger	*3* Slice the beef into long thin strips and add to the marinade. Cover and leave to marinate in the refrigerator for 2 hours.
Pepper, to taste	
1½ pounds strip loin steak	
1 red bell pepper	*4* Remove the stalk and seeds from the red bell pepper, and slice it into long strips. Set aside.
2 cups water	
1 cup basmati rice	*5* Pour the marinated beef through a sieve, and collect the liquid for use later.
1 tablespoon peanut oil	
1 cup broccolini	*6* In a large saucepan over high heat, add the water and basmati rice and bring to a boil. Turn down the heat, and simmer for 12 to 15 minutes, until all the water is absorbed and the rice is cooked well.
6 scallions	
1 tablespoon palm sugar	
2 tablespoons whole chia seeds	*7* Meanwhile, in a large wok, heat the oil over high heat. Add the beef, along with the chilies, garlic, and ginger collected in the sieve, and cook for 3 minutes, stirring often. Add the bell pepper and broccolini and cook for another 2 minutes. Chop the scallions into 1-inch pieces and add to the wok along with the palm sugar to cook for another 1 minute. Add the reserved marinade and simmer everything together for 2 to 3 minutes. Add the chia and give everything a good stir. Add more pepper if desired and serve immediately with the cooked rice.

Per serving: Calories 574 (From Fat 161); Fat 18g (Saturated 0g); Cholesterol 116mg; Sodium 1,196mg; Carbohydrate 59g (Dietary Fiber 5g); Protein 46g.

Roast Pork Steak with Chia Stuffing

Prep time: 10 min • **Cook time:** 30 min • **Yield:** 6 servings

Ingredients	Directions
6 strips bacon	*1* Preheat the oven to 375 degrees.
2 tablespoons olive oil	
1 onion, finely diced	*2* In a large frying pan, add 3 strips of the bacon and fry for 30 seconds each side. Remove the bacon, chop roughly, and set aside.
1 Granny Smith apple, grated	
Several sprigs rosemary, finely chopped	*3* Add 1 tablespoon of the olive oil to the pan, heat gently, and add the onion; cook for 10 minutes. Add the apple, rosemary, thyme, chia, breadcrumbs, and chopped bacon to the pan and mix well to combine everything evenly. Set aside.
1 bunch thyme, finely chopped	
4 tablespoons whole chia seeds	
1 cup breadcrumbs	
1 large pork steak (approximately 2 pounds)	*4* Clean the pork steak well. Make a horizontal slit to open it up and flatten it out, making sure not to cut all the way through.
8 medium potatoes, peeled	*5* Spread the stuffing out along the flattened pork steak and roll it up tightly. Wrap the 3 remaining strips of bacon around the pork steak to keep it together. You may need to use wooden skewers to keep everything together. Place the pork steak in a roasting tray and bake in the oven for 45 to 55 minutes.
3 carrots, peeled and chopped into 1-inch pieces	
2 parsnips, peeled and chopped into 1-inch pieces	
Salt and pepper, to taste	
	6 In a large saucepan, boil some water and add the potatoes to cook for 4 to 5 minutes. Drain and shake the pot a little to fluff up the potatoes and lay them out on a large baking sheet along with the carrots and parsnips. Drizzle with the remaining 1 tablespoon of oil, season with salt and pepper, and place in the oven to cook for 45 minutes. Serve the roast pork steak immediately with the roasted vegetables.

Per serving: Calories 668 (From Fat 246); Fat 27g (Saturated 8g); Cholesterol 99mg; Sodium 452mg; Carbohydrate 72g (Dietary Fiber 11g); Protein 35g.

Chicken Red Curry with Chia

Prep time: 20 min • **Cook time:** 20 min • **Yield:** 4 servings

Ingredients	Directions
1 pound skinless, boneless chicken thighs	**1** Chop the chicken thighs into bite-size pieces.
One 15-ounce can full-fat coconut milk	**2** In a bowl, put the coconut milk and mix well using a fork. Set aside.
1 cup basmati rice	**3** In a large saucepan, put the rice and water and bring to a boil. Reduce the heat and simmer for 12 to 15 minutes, until all the water is absorbed and the rice is cooked well.
2 cups water	
1 tablespoon vegetable oil	
½ red chili, thinly chopped	**4** Meanwhile, in a large wok, heat the vegetable oil over high heat and fry the chili and garlic for 1 minute; then add the curry paste.
3 cloves garlic, thinly chopped	
2 tablespoons red curry paste	**5** Add 1 ladle of coconut milk to the paste and stir well; cook for 2 minutes.
1 red bell pepper, thinly sliced	**6** Add the chicken pieces and cook for 5 minutes.
½ head broccoli, cut into small pieces	**7** Add the red bell pepper and broccoli and cook for 4 minutes.
6 scallions, thinly chopped	
Zest and juice of 1 lime	**8** Add the scallions and cook for 2 minutes.
½ cup chicken stock	**9** Add the juice and zest of the lime, the chicken stock, the remaining coconut milk, the soy sauce, the fish sauce, and the palm sugar and cook for 3 minutes, stirring often.
3 tablespoons light soy sauce	
1 tablespoon fish sauce	
1 tablespoon palm sugar	
2 tablespoons whole chia seeds	**10** Remove from the heat, add the chia, and stir well to combine.
	11 Serve immediately with the cooked rice.

Per serving: Calories 688 (From Fat 333); Fat 37g (Saturated 23g); Cholesterol 106mg; Sodium 1,143mg; Carbohydrate 68g (Dietary Fiber 8g); Protein 29g.

Chia Meatballs

Prep time: 15 min • **Cook time:** 30 min • **Yield:** 6 servings

Ingredients	Directions
2 tablespoons olive oil	*1* Preheat the oven to 400 degrees. Line a baking sheet with parchment paper.
½ onion, peeled and finely chopped	*2* In a large frying pan, heat the oil over medium heat.
1 garlic clove, peeled and crushed	*3* Add the onion to the pan, and cook for 4 minutes.
2 tablespoons tomato puree	*4* Add the garlic to the pan, and cook for 2 minutes.
2 eggs	*5* Add the tomato puree to the pan, and cook another 2 minutes, stirring continuously.
½ cup grated cheddar cheese	
1 pound ground beef	*6* Remove the pan from the heat and allow to cool a little.
½ cup breadcrumbs	*7* In a large bowl, beat the eggs; then add the beaten eggs and all the remaining ingredients to the frying pan.
2 tablespoons milled chia seeds	
1 teaspoon salt	*8* Mix with clean hands until well combined.
3 tablespoons finely chopped oregano	*9* Form the mixture into 18 meatballs measuring around 2 inches in diameter.
3 tablespoons finely chopped parsley	*10* Lay the meatballs out on the baking sheet.
3 tablespoons hot sauce	*11* Bake for 15 to 18 minutes until cooked through.
	12 Turn the meatballs occasionally, making sure they don't burn underneath.

Per serving: Calories 292 (From Fat 167); Fat 19g (Saturated 7g); Cholesterol 120mg; Sodium 801mg; Carbohydrate 11g (Dietary Fiber 2g); Protein 21g.

Tip: These meatballs are great served on a bed of rice with some sour cream and salsa on the side.

Lamb and Chia Tagine

Prep time: 25 min • **Cook time:** 1 hr 30 min • **Yield:** 8 servings

Ingredients	Directions
1 teaspoon ground cumin	**1** Preheat the oven to 350 degrees.
1 teaspoon ground cilantro	
¼ teaspoon ground turmeric	**2** In a small bowl, mix the cumin, ground cilantro, turmeric, pepper, and flour. Toss the meat in this flour mixture.
1 teaspoon pepper	
2 tablespoons flour	
1½ pounds diced lamb	**3** In a large ovenproof casserole dish or Dutch oven, heat 2 tablespoons of the oil over medium heat and brown the lamb in batches, adding more oil when needed. Remove the lamb and set aside.
4 tablespoons olive oil	
1 onion, diced	
3 garlic cloves, finely chopped	**4** Add 1 tablespoon of the oil to the dish; add the onion and cook for 5 to 6 minutes. Add the garlic, chili, and ginger. Chop the stalks off the cilantro and add half the leaves to the dish. Toss everything together so it's well coated in the oil; return the lamb to the dish.
1 red chili, deseeded and sliced	
One 3-inch piece fresh ginger, peeled and grated	
1 small bunch fresh cilantro	**5** Peel and dice the carrots, parsnips, and turnip into 1-inch cubes; add to the dish and cook for 4 to 5 minutes.
2 carrots	
2 parsnips	
½ turnip	**6** Add the water, sugar, raisins, and tomatoes and bring to a boil for 5 minutes.
4 cups water	
1 tablespoon dark brown sugar	**7** Cover the dish and place in the oven for 1 hour, checking occasionally to see if it needs more water. Remove from the oven, and add the chia. Stir the remaining cilantro through the dish and serve.
1 handful raisins	
½ a 15-ounce can chopped tomatoes	
2 tablespoons whole chia seeds	

Per serving: Calories 328 (From Fat 112); Fat 13g (Saturated 3g); Cholesterol 57mg; Sodium 139mg; Carbohydrate 33g (Dietary Fiber 5g); Protein 21g.

Seafood Dinners

Fresh fish makes a great meal. All you have to do with most types of good-quality fresh fish is fry it in a little olive oil, and it makes a great supper. To add chia, simply sprinkle some whole seeds over your cooked fish. Fish is a great source of omega-3 fatty acids, so when you add chia to your fish dinners you get a double-whammy hit of omega-3s that your heart, mind, and body will thank you for.

When you're choosing fresh fish, follow these tips:

- Look for bright, clear eyes.
- The gills should be a rich red.
- It shouldn't have a fishy smell — it should smell of the sea.
- Skin should look shiny and clean, not dull or discolored.
- If there is liquid around the fish, it should be clear, not milky.
- If you press the flesh, your fingerprint should quickly disappear, not linger.

In this section, we give you a taste of what can be done with fish other than just enjoying it freshly cooked from the pan.

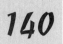

Easy Fish Pie

Prep time: 30 min • **Cook time:** 1 hr 10 min • **Yield:** 8 servings

Ingredients	Directions
3 pounds potatoes, peeled	*1* Preheat the oven to 325 degrees. Bring a large saucepan of salted water to a boil. Add the potatoes to the boiling water; simmer for 8 to 12 minutes. You want them to be just cooked through but still intact and not falling apart. Drain and allow the potatoes to dry. Mash the potatoes, adding ½ cup of the milk and 1 tablespoon of the butter. Season with salt and pepper; set aside.
3 cups 2 percent milk	
2 tablespoons butter	
Salt and pepper, to taste	
4 eggs	
1 pound white fish such as cod, monkfish, or plaice	*2* In a saucepan of boiling water, boil the eggs for 10 minutes until hard-boiled; allow the eggs to cool, and then remove the shells. Set aside.
½ pound fresh salmon	
½ pound smoked haddock	*3* In a large saucepan, add the remaining 2½ cups of the milk and bring to a boil over medium heat. Add all the fish to the simmering milk and simmer gently for 5 minutes. Remove the pieces of fish with a slotted spoon and set aside. Pour the milk through a sieve and collect the fish-flavored milk in a bowl.
1 tablespoon olive oil	
1 zucchini, sliced	
3 scallions, chopped	
1 tablespoon flour	*4* In a frying pan, heat the olive oil over medium heat; add the zucchini and cook gently for 5 to 6 minutes. Add the chopped scallions and cook for another 1 minute. Toss the vegetables onto some paper towels to absorb the excess oil; set aside.
1 tablespoon Dijon mustard	
Zest of 1 lemon	
2 tablespoons milled chia seeds	
	5 In a medium saucepan, melt the remaining 1 tablespoon of butter. Add the flour, fish-flavored milk, mustard, and lemon zest and bring to a boil.
	6 To assemble the pie, lay the fish pieces on the bottom of a 9-x-13-inch baking dish. Cut the eggs into quarter segments and toss over the fish along with the chia and vegetables. Then pour the sauce over evenly. Spread the mashed potatoes over everything and bake in the oven for 1 hour.

Per serving: Calories 377 (From Fat 101); Fat 11g (Saturated 4g); Cholesterol 165mg; Sodium 473mg; Carbohydrate 37g (Dietary Fiber 4g); Protein 32g.

Samui Prawns

Prep time: 15 min • **Cook time:** 10 min • **Yield:** 4 servings

Ingredients	Directions
2 cups rice noodles	*1* Bring a medium saucepan of salted water to a boil and add the rice noodles. Simmer the noodles for 3 minutes or according to package instructions. Drain in a colander and allow the noodles to dry. Set aside.
3 tablespoons peanut oil	
2 cups raw tiger prawns, peeled and deveined	
6 cloves garlic, peeled and roughly chopped	*2* In a large wok, heat the peanut oil over high heat.
One 3-inch piece fresh ginger, peeled and cut into match-stick-size pieces	*3* Add the prawns and cook for 2 minutes.
3 bird's-eye chilies, cut in half horizontally	*4* Add the garlic, ginger, and chilies and cook for 1 minute.
1 head bok choy, thinly sliced horizontally	*5* Add the bok choy, bell pepper, and sugar snap peas and cook for 1 minute, turning occasionally.
1 red bell pepper, thinly sliced	
½ cup sugar snap peas, cut lengthwise at an angle	*6* Add the soy sauce, fish sauce, palm sugar, basil, and plenty of pepper. Stir-fry for another 2 minutes.
3 tablespoons light soy sauce	
1 tablespoon fish sauce	*7* Add the cooked noodles to the wok and give everything a good stir. Cook for another 2 minutes and remove from the heat.
1 tablespoon palm sugar	
1 bunch basil, finely chopped	*8* Add the chia and stir again. Serve immediately.
Pepper, to taste	
2 tablespoons whole chia seeds	

Per serving: Calories 302 (From Fat 117); Fat 13g (Saturated 2g); Cholesterol 114mg; Sodium 1,346mg; Carbohydrate 29g (Dietary Fiber 5g); Protein 18g.

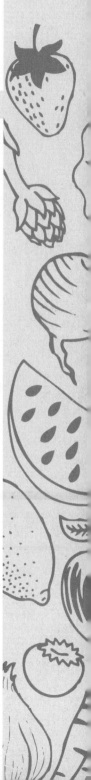

Pan-Fried Salmon and Creamy Chia Cabbage

Prep time: 15 min • **Cook time:** 15 min • **Yield:** 4 servings

Ingredients	Directions
½ **large savoy cabbage, chopped**	*1* Bring a large saucepan of water to a boil over high heat. Add the cabbage and cook for 1 minute. Drain through a colander and rinse with cold running water. Drain again and set aside to dry, using paper towels to dab away any excess liquid.
2 tablespoons olive oil	
1 onion, finely diced	
1 tablespoon white wine vinegar	*2* In a large frying pan, heat 1 tablespoon of the oil over high heat. Add the onion and cook for 5 minutes. Add the cabbage and cook for another 3 minutes. Add the vinegar and cook for another 1 minute, until evaporated. Add the wine and cook until reduced by half. Stir in the cream, bring to a boil, and season to taste. Remove from the heat and stir in the chia until well incorporated. Add the chives and parsley and stir well. Cover and keep warm.
⅓ cup dry white wine	
½ cup full-fat cream	
1 tablespoon milled chia seeds	
1 tablespoon chopped fresh chives	
1 tablespoon chopped fresh parsley	*3* In a separate large frying pan, heat the remaining 1 tablespoon of oil over medium heat. Add the salmon and cook for 3 minutes on each side, until the fish is cooked through. Season with salt and pepper.
4 salmon filets	
Salt and pepper, to taste	
	4 Serve the cooked salmon with the still-warm creamy chia cabbage.

Per serving: Calories 587 (From Fat 283); Fat 32g (Saturated 10g); Cholesterol 178mg; Sodium 402mg; Carbohydrate 10g (Dietary Fiber 3g); Protein 64g.

Shellfish Spaghetti with Chia

Prep time: 20 min • **Cook time:** 20 min • **Yield:** 4 servings

Ingredients	Directions
2 pounds fresh mussels, debearded	**1** Wash the mussels thoroughly and discard any shells that are open or broken (they aren't fresh and are unsafe to eat).
3 large tomatoes	
1 pound spaghetti	**2** Cut X's into the bottom of the tomatoes and put them in boiling water for a few minutes to soften. Remove the skins and the seeds from the tomatoes and chop the flesh into small cubes. Set aside.
1 cup raw prawns, shelled and deveined	
1 onion, peeled and thinly sliced	**3** Bring a large saucepan of salted water to a boil and cook the spaghetti for 8 to 10 minutes or according to the package instructions.
1 cup dry white wine	
Juice of 1 lemon	**4** In a separate large saucepan, place the cleaned mussels. Add the prawns, onion, and wine. Bring to a boil over high heat; then simmer for 5 minutes. Remove from the heat and drain, reserving the cooking liquid in a saucepan. Discard any unopened mussels.
2 sprigs fresh tarragon, stalks removed	
¼ cup full-fat cream	
2 tablespoons whole chia seeds	**5** Add the lemon juice to the pan of reserved cooking water. Bring the saucepan of cooking water to a boil over high heat and simmer until it reduces by half.
Salt and pepper, to taste	
	6 Cut the tarragon leaves into strips and add to the liquid. Stir in the cream.
	7 Add the tomatoes to the sauce, stir, and cook for another 2 minutes.
	8 Add the mussels, prawns, and drained spaghetti to the sauce and stir.
	9 Add the chia, stir well to combine, and season with salt and pepper. Serve immediately.

Per serving: Calories 653 (From Fat 109); Fat 12g (Saturated 5g); Cholesterol 96mg; Sodium 613mg; Carbohydrate 101g (Dietary Fiber 9g); Protein 33g.

Sides and Sauces

Side dishes and sauces can be what makes good dinners great. What people remember about a meal may be the sauce you served with that steak or the vegetable side dish that was to die for. The extras make a meal memorable. Plus, they can help bulk up a meal and provide more nutrients. By adding chia to your side dishes and sauces, you can add the extra nutrients without affecting the flavor.

In this section, we include recipes for ratatouille and samosas to serve on the side. Because chilies are used in so many sauces for heat, we've included a recipe for chia seed chili sauce that you can use at any meal.

Following is a ranking of the heat of common chili peppers. The scale is from 0 to 10, with 10 being the hottest:

Chili Pepper	*Heat*
Amarillo	4–5
Anaheim	2–3
Bird's eye	7–9
Cayenne	6–7
Chipotle	6–10
Habanero	8–9
Jalapeño	5–7
Poblano	3
Scotch bonnet	10
Serrano	7
Thai	6–7

Chia Ratatouille

Prep time: 30 min • **Cook time:** 1 hr • **Yield:** 8 servings

Ingredients	*Directions*
1 eggplant	*1* Preheat the oven to 350 degrees.
Salt, to taste	
2 onions	*2* Cut the eggplant in half lengthways; then slice it into 1-inch chunks. Lay out all the pieces of eggplant and sprinkle them generously with salt; allow them to sit for at least an hour.
3 garlic cloves	
1 red bell pepper	
1 yellow bell pepper	*3* Peel the onions and chop them in quarters and then into eight chunks. Peel and crush the garlic. Remove the stalks and seeds from the bell peppers and roughly chop into bite-size pieces. Wash and slice the zucchinis into 1-inch pieces.
2 zucchinis	
4 tomatoes	
2 tablespoons olive oil	
1 bunch thyme	*4* Cut X's into the bottom of the tomatoes and dip them into a medium bowl of boiling water and leave for a couple minutes. Remove the skin and seeds from the tomatoes and roughly chop. Set aside.
½ cup vegetable stock	
Salt and pepper, to taste	
2 tablespoons whole chia seeds	*5* In a large ovenproof casserole dish or Dutch oven, heat the olive oil over medium heat. Add the onions and cook for 6 minutes.
	6 Wipe off any visible excess salt from the eggplant and add the eggplant to the casserole dish; cook for 2 minutes. Add the zucchinis to the dish and cook for 2 minutes. Add the bell peppers and tomatoes to the dish and cook for another 2 minutes.
	7 Remove the woody stalks from the thyme and add it to the dish. Give everything a good stir, add the vegetable stock, season with salt and pepper, and cook in the oven for 40 minutes.
	8 Remove from the oven, add the chia, and stir well.

Per serving: Calories 115 (From Fat 43); Fat 5g (Saturated 1g); Cholesterol 0mg; Sodium 302mg; Carbohydrate 17g (Dietary Fiber 5g); Protein 3g.

Vegetable Samosas

Prep time: 30 min • **Cook time:** 35 min • **Yield:** 8 servings

Ingredients	Directions
1 tablespoon tomato puree	*1* Preheat the oven to 375 degrees.
1 teaspoon garam masala	
1 teaspoon chili powder	*2* In a medium bowl, mix the tomato puree, garam masala, chili powder, ground cilantro, garlic, ginger, salt, yogurt, chopped cilantro, lemon juice, and water.
½ teaspoon ground cilantro	
2 cloves garlic, peeled and crushed	*3* Transfer everything from the bowl to a wok and cook over high heat for about 1 minute.
One 1-inch piece fresh ginger, peeled and grated	
Pinch of salt	*4* Add the mushrooms, bell pepper, carrot, and corn to the wok. Give everything a good stir and cook over low heat for 6 or 7 minutes, until everything is quite dry.
4 tablespoons plain yogurt	
1 tablespoon chopped fresh cilantro leaves	*5* Remove from the heat, add the chia, and stir well.
2 teaspoons lemon juice	
4 tablespoons water	*6* Working quickly with the filo pastry and using a plate or saucer as a template, cut as many 5-inch rounds as possible from each sheet of pastry.
5 mushrooms, thinly sliced	
½ red bell pepper, deseeded and diced	*7* Oil each round lightly and arrange 3 rounds on top of each other.
1 carrot, peeled and diced small	
2 tablespoons sweet corn	*8* Put about ⅛ of the vegetable mixture to one side of the pastry round and fold over the pastry in half to make a semicircle. Seal the edges by folding a tiny bit in from the edge so it doubles or triples itself; pinch down firmly. Brush the outside of the parcel lightly with oil.
2 tablespoons whole chia seeds	
12 sheets phyllo per conventions pastry	
2 tablespoons peanut oil	*9* Repeat with the remaining 7 samosas. Transfer to the oven to bake for 25 minutes or until golden brown.

Per serving: Calories 148 (From Fat 55); Fat 6g (Saturated 1g); Cholesterol 1mg; Sodium 183mg; Carbohydrate 20g (Dietary Fiber 2g); Protein 4g.

Chia Seed Chili Sauce

Prep time: 15 min • **Cook time:** 25 min • **Yield:** 24 servings

Ingredients	Directions
6 red chilies	**1** Tear the chilies roughly into quarters and remove the seeds, but reserve them for use later.
1 cup water	
¼ teaspoon ground allspice	**2** In a small saucepan, bring the water to a boil and add the torn chilies. Simmer for 5 minutes, until softened. Remove from the heat and allow to cool.
¼ teaspoon pepper	
⅛ teaspoon ground cinnamon	**3** In a medium saucepan, combine the reserved chili seeds, allspice, pepper, and cinnamon over medium heat for 2 to 3 minutes, until the seeds are lightly toasted.
2 large tomatoes	
¼ cup whole chia seeds	
2 garlic cloves, peeled and minced	**4** Cut X's into the bottoms of the tomatoes. Put the tomatoes in a bowl of boiling water and allow to sit for a few minutes, until the skins soften. Remove the skins and the seeds from the tomatoes. Chop the tomatoes roughly.
¼ teaspoon salt	
3 cups chicken stock	
	5 In a blender, put the chilies and the water they were cooked in. Add to the blender the chili seed and spice mixture, the chopped tomatoes, and the chia. Blend for 1 or 2 minutes until well combined. Pour this puree back into the saucepan.
	6 Add the garlic, salt, and chicken stock to the saucepan. Bring to a boil over medium heat. Reduce the heat and simmer for 10 minutes or until the sauce has thickened. Stir the sauce often to prevent it from sticking.
	7 Serve the sauce immediately. Store any unused sauce in an airtight container in the refrigerator for up to 2 weeks.

**Per serving:** Calories 18 (From Fat 7); Fat 1g (Saturated 0g); Cholesterol 0mg; Sodium 143mg; Carbohydrate 2g (Dietary Fiber 1g); Protein 1g.

Chapter 11

Satisfying Dietary Restrictions

*W*hether by choice or because of an allergy or sensitivity, many people are restricted in the range of foods that they can consume. More and more people are opting for a vegetarian or vegan diet. And you can't go a day without hearing about the gluten-free diet. Other people have issues with dairy and either reducing or eliminating it from their diets. If you're on a restrictive diet, getting certain nutrients can be difficult, but because chia is dairy-free, gluten-free, and suitable for vegans and vegetarians, it offers great nutrition for everyone!

In this chapter, we give you recipes that are all about meeting specific dietary restrictions.

Vegetarian: Leaving Out the Meat

People all over the world decide not to consume meat, poultry, or seafood for a variety of reasons, including health, religion, and personal beliefs. A vegetarian diet can be beneficial to health if you make sure to meet your body's nutritional requirements. On average, vegetarians consume a lower proportion of calories from fat and generally have a lower body mass index (BMI), which has drawn more people to a plant-based diet.

Chia Quiche with Broccoli and Mushrooms

Prep time: 1 hr • **Cook time:** 45 min • **Yield:** 6 servings

Ingredients	*Directions*
1¾ cups whole-wheat pastry flour	*1* In a large bowl, sift the flour; add the milled chia seeds and salt. Add the sunflower oil and mix to combine. Add the water and mix into a soft dough.
¼ cup milled chia seeds	
¼ teaspoon salt	
⅓ cup sunflower oil	*2* On a worktop, sprinkle some flour and roll the dough to the desired thickness and shape.
⅓ cup water	
1 tablespoon extra-virgin olive oil	*3* Preheat the oven to 375 degrees.
¾ cup porcini mushrooms	*4* In a large frying pan, heat the oil over medium heat. Add the mushrooms to the pan and cook for 6 to 8 minutes. Remove the mushrooms from the pan with a slotted spoon and place on paper towel to remove any excess liquid.
¾ cup white button mushrooms	
3 garlic cloves, minced	
1 tablespoon dry basil	*5* In a large bowl, place the cooked mushrooms and all the remaining ingredients and mix together. Leave for a few minutes, and stir to ensure a nice mix of ingredients.
1 cup broccoli, diced	
2¾ cups silken tofu, crumbled	
2 tablespoons vinegar	*6* In a 9-inch pie pan, place the dough at the bottom of the dish. Add the mushroom mixture. Bake for 45 minutes. Remove and serve.
2 tablespoons sunflower oil	
½ teaspoon sea salt	
½ cup chia gel (see the Note)	

Per serving: Calories 359 (From Fat 218); Fat 25g (Saturated 3g); Cholesterol 0mg; Sodium 329mg; Carbohydrate 28g (Dietary Fiber 7g); Protein 11g.

Note: To make ½ cup chia gel, mix 2 tablespoons whole chia seeds with ¾ cup water. Stir well and let sit for 20 minutes, stirring occasionally.

Spaghetti Alfredo

Prep time: 30 min • **Cook time:** 30 min • **Yield:** 6 servings

Ingredients	Directions
½ **onion, chopped**	**1** In a pan on high heat, add the onion, green and red bell pepper, broccoli, celery, garlic, olive oil, and chia gel. Sauté until the vegetables are tender.
¼ **green bell pepper, chopped**	
¼ **red bell pepper, chopped**	
¼ **cup broccoli**	**2** Prepare the Alfredo sauce per the package instructions.
1 large celery stalk, chopped	
2 cloves garlic, minced	**3** Add the sauce to the pan of veggies and mix.
2 tablespoons olive oil	
½ **cup chia gel (see the Note)**	**4** Add the mushroom soup and water and mix.
One 10-ounce packet of Alfredo sauce	**5** Add the peas to the pan and cook on low heat for 3 minutes.
One 10-ounce can cream of mushroom soup	
1 cup of water	**6** Prepare the spaghetti per the package instructions.
¾ **cup frozen peas**	**7** When the spaghetti is ready, transfer it to a dish and pour the sauce on top.
1 pound spaghetti	
Basil and oregano, to taste	**8** Sprinkle with basil, oregano, and chia seeds.
1 teaspoon whole chia seeds	

Per serving: Calories 524 (From Fat 172); Fat 19g (Saturated 6g); Cholesterol 26mg; Sodium 774mg; Carbohydrate 71g (Dietary Fiber 7g); Protein 16g.

Note: To make ½ cup chia gel, mix 2 tablespoons whole chia seeds with ¾ cup water. Stir well and let sit for 20 minutes, stirring occasionally.

Vary It! Try changing up the vegetables you use. Add fresh chilies for a spicy kick! You can also try changing the pasta to capellini, penne, or linguine.

Vegetarian Pizza

Prep time: 20 min • **Cook time:** 30 min • **Yield:** 2 servings

Ingredients	Directions
¾ cup buckwheat flour	**1** In a bowl, mix the buckwheat flour, tapioca flour, and baking powder.
¼ cup tapioca flour	
1 teaspoon baking powder	**2** Add 2 tablespoons of the chia, the seasoning (if desired), and the salt and mix.
4 tablespoons whole chia seeds	
2 teaspoons seasoning of choice (optional)	**3** Add the yogurt and water and mix to achieve a light dough consistency.
½ teaspoon salt	**4** Preheat the oven to 400 degrees.
¾ cup soy yogurt	
¼ cup water	**5** On a floured surface, gently flatten the dough, pressing it into a large, thin circle. You should get approximately a 14- to 16-inch pizza.
⅔ cup tomato sauce	
1 cup mozzarella cheese	
¼ cup mushrooms	**6** Transfer the dough to a baking sheet and bake for 5 minutes. Remove the dough from the oven; let it cool.
¼ cup broccoli	
¼ cup olives	**7** In a small bowl, mix the remaining 2 tablespoons of chia seeds with the tomato sauce.
¼ cup hot peppers	
	8 Spread the sauce on the pizza dough base.
	9 Add the cheese, mushrooms, broccoli, olives, and hot peppers to the pizza.
	10 Bake for 15 to 20 minutes, keeping an eye on the pizza to ensure that it doesn't burn.

Per serving: Calories 580 (From Fat 231); Fat 26g (Saturated 9g); Cholesterol 44mg; Sodium 1,703mg; Carbohydrate 63g (Dietary Fiber 17g); Protein 27g.

Vary It! You can add or remove from this recipe whatever toppings you like. Just mix and match to get your favorite pizza!

Chia-Spiked Vegetarian Stir-Fry

Prep time: 20 min • **Cook time:** 15 min • **Yield:** 4 servings

Ingredients	Directions
3 large garlic cloves, finely chopped	*1* In a large wok or skillet on medium heat, sauté the garlic and ginger in the olive oil and sesame oil for 30 seconds.
2 teaspoons ginger root, finely grated	
½ teaspoon olive oil	*2* Add the soy sauce, vinegar, and water and stir-fry for another 30 seconds.
½ teaspoon sesame oil	
3 tablespoons soy sauce	*3* Add the kale, carrots, broccoli, onion, red and yellow bell peppers, mushrooms, and tomatoes; cover and cook, stirring occasionally.
3 tablespoons rice vinegar	
¾ cup water	
2 cups kale, chopped	*4* In about 10 minutes, when the vegetables are tender, remove from heat and add the whole chia seeds stirring to combine well.
2 carrots, chopped	
1 cup, broccoli	*5* Put the rice on a plate, and add the stir-fry to serve.
⅓ red onion, chopped	
⅓ red bell pepper, chopped	
⅓ yellow bell pepper, chopped	
1 cup mushrooms	
2 tomatoes, chopped	
3 tablespoons whole chia seeds	
5 cups cooked basmati rice	

Per serving: Calories 437 (From Fat 38); Fat 4g (Saturated 1g); Cholesterol 0mg; Sodium 744mg; Carbohydrate 95g (Dietary Fiber 8g); Protein 11g.

Vegan: Avoiding All Animal Products

A vegan diet is more restrictive than any of the vegetarian diets (see the nearby sidebar). Vegans don't eat any animal products or by-products. This includes the obvious — meat, fish, poultry, eggs, and dairy — as well as the less obvious (for example, honey, refined sugar, anything made with gelatin, and more). People who choose to be vegans usually do so for health, environmental, and/or ethical reasons. The key to a good vegan diet is eating a variety of fruits and vegetables, plenty of leafy greens, whole-grain products, nuts, and seeds.

Vegans don't eat fish, but chia can provide much-needed omega-3 fatty acids that are essential for heart health, memory, and many other body functions. Chia is among the best sources of plant-based omega-3s in the world, so it's perfect for people who don't eat fish.

Chia is also a *complete protein,* meaning that it has all nine essential amino acids that are required for building and repairing body cells. Usually, we need to get complete proteins from meat and animal products because high-quality protein is rare in the plant kingdom. But by adding chia to their diets, vegans don't miss out on this essential nutrient.

Finally, chia can be used as an egg replacement (see Chapter 5). Because vegans don't eat eggs, chia can come to the rescue and provide vegans with a binding agent that's suitable for their diets so they don't miss out on recipes that call for eggs.

TECHNICAL STUFF

Different strokes for different folks

Vegetarians fall into several categories:

- **Lacto-ovo vegetarians** don't eat meat, fish, and poultry, but they do eat dairy products and eggs.

- **Lacto vegetarians** don't eat meat, fish, poultry, and eggs, but they do eat dairy products.

- **Ovo vegetarians** don't eat meat, fish, poultry, or dairy products, but they do eat eggs.

- **Pescetarians** are like lacto-ovo vegetarians, except they eat seafood — in other words, they avoid meat and poultry, but they do eat seafood, dairy products, and eggs.

Got that straight?

Vegan Vanilla Chia Seed Pudding

Prep time: 1 hr 15 min • **Yield:** 8 servings

Ingredients	Directions
8 cups vanilla-flavored almond milk	**1** In a blender, add the almond milk, vanilla, and maple syrup and blend.
4 teaspoons vanilla extract	
4 tablespoons pure maple syrup	**2** Set the blender to a very low setting, add the chia, and blend.
1½ cups whole chia seeds	**3** Transfer the mixture to a bowl and give it a stir.
1 tablespoon shredded coconut	**4** Let sit for 5 minutes and stir again.
¼ cup goji berries	**5** Let sit for 5 more minutes and stir again.
¼ cup blueberries	**6** Add the coconut and stir.
	7 Add the goji berries and blueberries and stir.
	8 Pour the mixture into a container, such as a small glass jar, and place in the refrigerator for at least 4 hours or overnight.

Per serving: Calories 276 (From Fat 114); Fat 13g (Saturated 1g); Cholesterol 0mg; Sodium 162mg; Carbohydrate 35g (Dietary Fiber 12g); Protein 7g.

Vary It! Try adding cinnamon or ginger instead of vanilla. If you're not a fan of coconut, use orange or lemon peel. And change up the berries with whichever berries you like best.

Vegan Chia Coconut Bread

Prep time: 20 min • **Cook time:** 50 min • **Yield:** 8 servings

Ingredients	Directions
1 tablespoon milled chia seeds	**1** In a large bowl, add the milled chia seeds and water and stir. Let sit for approximately 15 minutes.
3 tablespoons water	
2 cups flour	**2** Preheat the oven to 350 degrees.
1 cup unrefined sugar	**3** In a large bowl, sift the flour; add the sugar, baking powder, baking soda, and salt and mix well.
1 teaspoon baking powder	
½ teaspoon baking soda	
½ teaspoon salt	**4** Add the bananas, coconut milk, coconut oil, and vanilla extract to the bowl of milled chia and water and combine all the ingredients together.
3 ripe bananas, mashed	
½ cup refrigerated coconut milk	
½ cup unrefined virgin coconut oil	**5** Create a well in the dry ingredients, and pour the wet ingredients in the center. Mix until all the ingredients are well combined.
1 teaspoon vanilla extract	
½ cup unsweetened shredded coconut	**6** Add the coconut to the mixture and combine again.
1 teaspoon whole chia seeds	**7** Pour the mixture into a greased loaf pan.
	8 Sprinkle the whole chia seeds on top of the mixture.
	9 Bake for 50 minutes or until a knife sliced into the center comes out clean.

Per serving: Calories 416 (From Fat 160); Fat 18g (Saturated 15g); Cholesterol 0mg; Sodium 278mg; Carbohydrate 60g (Dietary Fiber 3g); Protein 4g.

Vegan Salad and Chia Dressing

Prep time: 30 min • **Yield:** 2 servings

Ingredients	Directions
1 medium zucchini, spiraled	**1** In a large bowl, combined the zucchini, carrots, bell pepper, and cabbage, and toss with your hands.
2 large carrots, shredded	
1 red bell pepper, thinly sliced	**2** Top with the tofu, onions, chia seeds, and sesame seeds.
1 cup thinly sliced red cabbage	
¾ cup baked tofu (whatever flavor you like)	**3** Divide between two plates, and divide the Chia Dressing between the two plates.
3 green onions, thinly sliced	
1 tablespoon whole chia seeds	
1 teaspoon sesame seeds	
Chia Dressing (see the following recipe)	

Chia Dressing

Ingredients	Directions
1 tablespoon milled chia seeds	**1** In a blender, combine all the ingredients and blend on high until smooth.
3 tablespoons coconut milk	
½ tablespoon nutritional yeast	**2** Refrigerate for 10 minutes before serving to thicken the dressing.
½ tablespoon fresh lemon juice	
¼ teaspoon crushed garlic	
¼ teaspoon chili powder	
Pinch of sea salt	

Per serving: Calories 371 (From Fat 166); Fat 18g (Saturated 6g); Cholesterol 0mg; Sodium 512mg; Carbohydrate 28g (Dietary Fiber 11g); Protein 26g.

Saying "No, Thanks" to Gluten

One of the fastest-growing sectors in any supermarket is the gluten-free aisle, thanks to the massive influx of gluten-free products that manufacturers are coming up with as they try to meet consumer demand. *Gluten* is a protein complex found in wheat, barley, and rye, and lately, more people are actively avoiding it in their diets.

The big shift to gluten-free is due to a few factors:

- ✔ More people are being diagnosed with celiac disease, a disorder of the small intestine. People with celiac disease are prescribed a gluten-free diet.

- ✔ Some people choose to go gluten-free because they suffer allergic reactions to wheat, such as skin inflammation.

- ✔ Some people just avoid gluten because they believe it to be healthier.

Gluten intolerance is on the rise, and studies are being done to understand why this is the case. One reason may be the increased amount of gluten in our day-to-day diet — our ancestors didn't consume as much gluten, and some people's bodies may be unable to cope with this gluten consumption. Another reason may be that modern wheat, which is highly refined, is very different from the wheat that was available in our ancestors' day and has a lot more gluten.

Chia is naturally gluten-free and can be added to many recipes to help gluten-intolerant people get the nutrients they need. Plus, the milled form of chia can sometimes be used instead of flour, so it's a great alternative.

Gluten-Free Chia, Cranberry, and Coconut Granola

Prep time: 20 min • **Cook time:** 30 min • **Yield:** 6 servings

Ingredients	Directions
6 cups old-fashioned gluten-free oats	**1** Preheat the oven to 325 degrees.
1¼ cups whole chia seeds	**2** In a large bowl, combine the oats, chia, coconut, and almonds.
1½ cups shredded coconut	
1½ cups almonds, chopped	**3** Mix in the brown sugar, ginger, cinnamon, and salt.
¼ cup brown sugar	
1 teaspoon ground ginger	**4** In a small saucepan, heat the coconut oil over medium heat for about 3 minutes, until it melts completely. Add it to the mixture.
2 teaspoons cinnamon	
1 teaspoon salt	
½ cup coconut oil	**5** Mix in the agave syrup and almond extract and mix it very well.
1 cup agave syrup	
1 teaspoon almond extract	**6** Spread the mixture onto a baking sheet.
2 egg whites	**7** Brush the mixture with the egg whites.
1½ cups dried cranberries	
	8 Bake for 10 minutes, remove from the oven, and stir on the baking sheet.
	9 Return to the oven for another 20 minutes or until golden brown.
	10 Remove from the oven and let it cool completely.
	11 Add the cranberries and transfer to an air-tight container.

Per serving: Calories 1,250 (From Fat 544); Fat 61g (Saturated 27g); Cholesterol 0mg; Sodium 484mg; Carbohydrate 163g (Dietary Fiber 27g); Protein 25g.

Vary It! You can add whatever berries you like, or try mixing more than one — such as raspberries and strawberries. You can make this granola vegan by leaving out the egg whites.

Gluten-Free Chia Pancakes

Prep time: 10 min • **Cook time:** 15 min • **Yield:** 8 servings

Ingredients	Directions
1 cup brown rice flour	*1* Heat a frying pan on low.
1 teaspoon baking powder	
A pinch of sea salt	*2* In a large bowl, add the brown rice flour, baking powder, and salt. Mix together.
½ banana	
1 tablespoon whole chia seeds	*3* On a plate, mash the banana; add the chia seeds and mix.
1 egg	
⅔ cup almond milk	*4* Add the banana and chia mixture to the dry mixture and combine.
1 teaspoon vanilla extract	
½ cup berries of your choice	*5* Add the egg, almond milk, and vanilla extract to the mixture. Mix well to ensure an even consistency.
Butter, for cooking	
	6 Add the berries to the batter and mix well.
	7 Add some butter to the pan and place ¼ cup of the batter onto the pan.
	8 Cook for 1 or 2 minutes.
	9 Flip and cook the other side, until brown.
	10 Repeat to make the remaining pancakes.

Per serving: Calories 116 (From Fat 29); Fat 3g (Saturated 1g); Cholesterol 27mg; Sodium 91mg; Carbohydrate 19g (Dietary Fiber 2g); Protein 3g.

Note: If you find it hard to get rice flour, you can use spelt flour. Just be sure to read the label to make sure it's gluten-free.

Vary It! Try adding fresh berries and maple syrup. Just make sure to read the label to make sure it's gluten-free.

Gluten-Free Chia Chicken Korma

Prep time: 15 min • **Cook time:** 30 min • **Yield:** 4 servings

Ingredients	Directions
1¼ cups uncooked rice	**1** Prepare a pot of boiling water and cook the rice per the package instructions.
3 tablespoons sunflower oil	
2 cardamom pods, crushed	**2** In a large pan over low heat, put the oil, cardamom, cinnamon, crushed cilantro, cumin, and turmeric; cook for 1 minute. Watch to make sure the spices don't burn.
1 teaspoon ground cinnamon	
1½ teaspoons cilantro, crushed	
1 teaspoon ground cumin	
2 teaspoons turmeric	**3** Add the onion and cook for about 3 minutes. Add the garlic and ginger, and cook for 1 or 2 minutes more.
1 onion, thinly chopped	
3 garlic cloves, chopped	
1 small fresh ginger piece, peeled and chopped	**4** Add the chicken, coat it in the spices, and cook for a few minutes.
4 chicken breasts, cut into small pieces	**5** Add the coconut milk and bring the liquid to a boil. Reduce the heat and let simmer for 8 to 12 minutes. The chicken will be tender and the liquid will reduce.
1¾ cups coconut milk	
½ cup plain yogurt	**6** Add the yogurt and cream to the mixture, making sure it doesn't boil.
½ cup heavy whipping cream	
¼ cup whole chia seeds	**7** Sprinkle the chia, almonds, and fresh cilantro over the mixture.
¼ cup flaked almonds	
½ cup fresh cilantro	**8** Serve the rice and add the korma either on the side or in the center of the rice.

Per serving: Calories 901 (From Fat 477); Fat 53g (Saturated 29g); Cholesterol 116mg; Sodium 120mg; Carbohydrate 69g (Dietary Fiber 7g); Protein 40g.

Note: Korma is a dish that originated in south or central Asia. It's usually made with yogurt, cream, nut and seed pastes, or coconut milk. It's often the less fiery choice of curry dish because it's usually made with less chilies, but it's still full of flavor.

Gluten-Free Apple Pie Chia Parfait Dessert

Prep time: 15 min • **Cook time:** 20 min • **Yield:** 4 servings

Ingredients	Directions
1 cup gluten-free rolled oats	**1** In a large bowl, combine the oats, 4 tablespoons of the whole chia seeds, the almond milk, 2 teaspoons of the vanilla extract, 1 teaspoon of the cinnamon, and the stevia and whisk to combine.
10 tablespoons whole chia seeds	
2½ cups almond milk	**2** Refrigerate for 4 hours. If you're not happy with the thickness, you can add almond milk to soften it or chia seeds to thicken it.
3 teaspoons vanilla extract	
2½ teaspoons cinnamon	**3** In a large pot, add the apples, apple juice, 4 tablespoons of the whole chia seeds, the remaining 1½ teaspoons of cinnamon, and the remaining 1 teaspoon of vanilla extract.
1 tablespoon stevia	
6 apples, peeled and diced	
1½ cups apple juice	**4** Bring to a low boil.
	5 Reduce the heat to medium-low and simmer for 15 minutes, stirring every few minutes.
	6 When the apples are tender by piercing with a knife, turn off the heat.
	7 Mash 50 percent of the mixture; set aside to cool.
	8 In 4 large cups or parfait glasses, layer the oats and then the jam in each, a few spoonfuls per layer. Continue layering until everything is used. Sprinkle the remaining 2 tablespoons of chia seeds on top of each parfait.

Per serving: Calories 388 (From Fat 103); Fat 12g (Saturated 1g); Cholesterol 0mg; Sodium 100mg; Carbohydrate 67g (Dietary Fiber 15g); Protein 8g.

Got Dairy? Nope

The main reason people avoid dairy is because they're *lactose intolerant,* which means they can't digest lactose. *Lactose* is the natural sugar in animal milks and dairy products made from animal milks. In the stomach, lactose needs to be broken down by a certain enzyme, and people who are lactose intolerant don't produce this enzyme. So, the undigested lactose remains in their stomachs and causes discomfort. The best way to deal with lactose intolerance is to cut out dairy products that contain lactose so that your body doesn't need to break down lactose.

Some people who are lactose intolerant can use dairy products that have had the lactose removed. If you fall into this group, be sure to read food labels to ensure that if you're using certain dairy products, they're lactose-free.

People who are lactose intolerant can use substitutes. Here are some examples of substitutes:

✔ **Butter:** Use soy margarine or coconut oil instead.

✔ **Cheese:** Use soy substitutes.

✔ **Milk:** Use soymilk or almond milk.

✔ **Chocolate with milk ingredients:** Use dairy-free dark chocolate.

Changing your cooking habits can be challenging. Avoiding milk, yogurt, and other easily recognized dairy products is simple enough, but you also have to be conscious of ingredients that are derived from dairy, such as butter, cream, cheese, casein (a binding agent), curd, whey, and whey proteins, because these are all dairy-related products.

Lactose-intolerant people aren't the only ones who need to use these substitutes. Many nutritionists and dietitians advise people to stay away from dairy altogether. Chia seeds are naturally dairy-free so whatever reasons you have for choosing to avoid dairy, this section gives you a few ideas on how to do so.

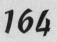

Dairy-Free Chocolate Chia Pudding

Prep time: 12–17 min • **Yield:** 4 servings

Ingredients	Directions
3 cups almond milk	*1* In a medium bowl, add the almond milk and cocoa powder; whisk to combine.
2 tablespoons unsweetened cocoa powder	
½ cup whole chia seeds	*2* Stir in the chia, vanilla extract, and stevia.
1 teaspoon vanilla extract	*3* Pour into 4 glasses and cool in the refrigerator for 10 to 15 minutes.
½ teaspoon stevia	
4 tablespoons coconut milk	*4* Pour 1 tablespoon of the coconut milk on each dessert before serving.

Per serving: *Calories 181 (From Fat 106); Fat 12g (Saturated 4g); Cholesterol 0mg; Sodium 116mg; Carbohydrate 17g (Dietary Fiber 9g); Protein 5g.*

Vary It! You can change this chia pudding recipe to include fresh fruits instead of chocolate.

Making your own almond milk

You can make your own almond milk from scratch if you don't want to buy store-bought milk. Here's how:

1. Soak ½ cup of raw almonds in a large bowl of water overnight.
2. Rinse the almonds well after soaking.
3. In a blender, combine the almonds, 2 cups of water, 1 tablespoon of pure maple syrup, 1 teaspoon of lemon juice, and ¼ teaspoon of salt. Blend on high for 1 or 2 minutes.
4. Pour the mixture into a fine mesh bag or a specialized nut bag over a large container.
5. Collect all the liquid in the container by squeezing the bag.

You can use this almond milk in lots of recipes calling for milk. It's even delicious on its own, served in a tall glass with ice.

Dairy-Free Mac and Cheese

Prep time: 10 min • **Cook time:** 10 min • **Yield:** 2 servings

Ingredients	Directions
2 cups uncooked elbow pasta	*1* In a large saucepan, bring salted water to a boil.
4 tablespoons dairy-free margarine	*2* Add the pasta and cook for 8 to 12 minutes or according to the package instructions.
¼ cup flour	
1½ cups rice milk	*3* In a medium saucepan, melt the margarine over low heat for 2 to 3 minutes.
1 cup dairy-free cheddar cheese	
½ teaspoon mustard powder	*4* Add the flour and whisk for 1 minute.
½ teaspoon salt	*5* Add 1 cup of the rice milk, whisking constantly until it comes to a boil. Continue to whisk for another 1 minute.
¼ teaspoon pepper	
2 tablespoons whole chia seeds, plus extra for garnish	*6* Add the cheese and stir with a wooden spoon for 3 to 5 minutes, until it's well combined.
	7 Add the remaining ½ cup of rice milk, along with the mustard powder, salt, pepper, and 2 tablespoons of the chia.
	8 Stir everything until the cheese has melted and a smooth consistency is attained.
	9 Add the cooked and drained pasta and stir well.
	10 Top with extra chia seeds.

Per serving: Calories 775 (From Fat 365); Fat 41g (Saturated 11g); Cholesterol 0mg; Sodium 1,262mg; Carbohydrate 88g (Dietary Fiber 6g); Protein 12g.

Note: Many dairy-free cheeses are available, but be sure to check the label and look out for casein, which is a milk protein. The best cheese alternatives that we've found are Daiya and WayFare, both of which are vegan. Daiya is available in mozzarella and cheddar flavors, and it melts beautifully and is fantastic on pizza. WayFare is a spreadable cheese product, perfect for sandwiches.

Chapter 12

Especially for Kids

In This Chapter

▶ Convincing your kids to eat well

▶ Supercharging your kids' favorite dinners

▶ Snacking on the healthy stuff

▶ Adding more nutrients to kids' sweet treats

*W*hen you're a parent, particularly of young kids, one of your daily worries is what has gone into their little bodies. Was it healthy? Have they eaten enough? Have they eaten too much sugar? Have they gotten enough vitamins? At the end of the day, as you turn out the lights, these questions are often still looming, but if you make sure that they eat chia every day, you can sleep a little easier, knowing that they've gotten omega-3 fatty acids, fiber, and high-quality protein, and they're well on their way to meeting their vitamin and mineral requirements.

Because chia is virtually taste-free, you can put it into your kids' meals without their suspecting a thing. So, even if you have picky eaters under your roof, you can make sure they get all the nutrition they need while they munch on their favorite foods.

Kids need good nutrition to fuel their growing bodies, so if you can manage to fill them with the right foods, they can get on with the more important tasks of having fun and growing up healthy. This chapter is all about tips and tricks for doing just that. We give you recipes that your kids will love.

Getting a Great Start

One of the most vital things you can do as a parent is teach your children healthy eating habits. Offering them healthy, tasty foods that they love and want more of will help ensure that they go on to make healthy food choices as adults. If you can encourage your children to eat a balanced diet throughout their school years, you're giving them the best possible chance of staying healthy throughout their lives.

Learning the importance of nutrition at a young age

A balanced diet has the right mix of carbohydrates, fats, protein, vitamins, and minerals. Adults are encouraged to eat a high-fiber, low-fat diet, but kids have very different nutritional needs. At different stages, they need more fat in their diets than adults need, and their tiny tummies need to take in higher concentrations of calories and nutrients to support growth and development. Chances are, your little ones won't care much about any of this, but they will care how it tastes — so you need to provide nutritious meals that are tasty, too!

The sooner kids become aware that what they're eating is what fuels their bodies, the better. A good way to start explaining the importance of nutrition is to try to encourage kids to eat a variety of different colored foods. Different colored fruits and vegetables provide different essential nutrients, so they help in the quest for balance.

As your kids get a bit older, bring them grocery shopping to show them what you buy to make healthy dinners. That way, they'll get to know the difference between the healthy and unhealthy convenience foods available. More important, they'll know what to shop for when they grow up.

Encourage your kids to learn the differences between healthy and unhealthy fats, what carbohydrates are good for us, and what foods are full of hidden sugars. You can do this by reading books and playing games that encourage healthy eating. Make sure your children know the results of a bad diet, such as poor health. The aim is that by educating children about healthy food choices at home, it will encourage them to eat well when they're outside the home.

Getting kids involved in the kitchen

Kids who play a part in making their own food have a much better chance of eating that food, so if you have fussy eaters at home, try getting them involved a bit more. Buy some fun aprons, wash their hands, and let them dive into home cooking. Kids love to mix, roll, measure out ingredients, and generally get their hands dirty in the kitchen.

A great way to start is by letting them make faces on dishes such as pizza. Using tomatoes for eyes, sliced peppers for mouths, mushrooms for ears, and broccoli for noses help make meals into playtime. Let your kids design their own dishes, and they'll be asking to do more next time.

Try to get them involved as much as possible with every step of the meal-prep process. When you're chopping vegetables, take out an extra chopping board and arm your little one with a blunt knife (one they can't hurt themselves with) and let them chop alongside you. These early cooking experiences will help encourage lifelong habits and make great family memories.

Favorite Dinners

Fussy eaters often go back to the same foods again and again, so to encourage healthy eating, a good place to start is with their favorite dinners. Chia will go unnoticed in most dishes so start with their favorites before moving on to more nutritious foods.

The recipes in this section are classic kid dinners that are not only economical but also healthy.

Lasagne

Prep time: 30 min • **Cook time:** 1 hr • **Yield:** 8 servings

Ingredients	Directions
1½ pounds lean ground beef	**1** In a large frying pan, cook the beef over medium-high heat for approximately 20 minutes until cooked through. Drain off any excess liquid.
2 tablespoons olive oil	
1 onion, finely chopped	
2 cloves garlic, crushed	**2** In a separate large frying pan, heat the oil over medium heat. Add the onion and cook for 10 minutes, until soft. Add the garlic and mushrooms to the frying pan with the onions.
1 cup sliced mushrooms	
1 zucchini	
One 15-ounce can chopped tomatoes	**3** Cut the zucchini lengthways twice, so you have four longs strips, and then slice those strips into ½-inch cubes. Add the zucchini to the vegetables, and cook for another 6 to 8 minutes.
½ teaspoon sugar	
3 tablespoons tomato puree	
1 vegetable bouillon cube	**4** When the beef is cooked through, add it to the vegetables. Add the chopped tomatoes, sugar, and tomato puree; mix well.
1 tablespoon balsamic vinegar	
1 teaspoon dried oregano	**5** Dissolve the vegetable bouillon cube in ½ cup boiling water, and add it to the pan with the meat and vegetables.
½ teaspoon pepper	
2 tablespoons butter	
2 tablespoons flour	**6** Add the vinegar, oregano, and pepper to the pan. Mix everything together well, turn down the heat, and let simmer for another 20 minutes, stirring occasionally.
1½ cups 2 percent milk	
Salt, to taste	
Ground white pepper, to taste	**7** Meanwhile, in a medium saucepan, melt the butter over medium heat. Remove from the heat and add the flour to the saucepan with the butter. Mix well, until the flour is well absorbed, and cook for 1 minute. Add the milk gradually, stirring continuously. Add the salt and ground white pepper.
4 tablespoons whole chia seeds	
½ teaspoon salt	
12 dry lasagna sheets	
2 cups grated cheddar cheese	

8 Bring the milk and flour mixture to a boil, stirring continuously with a whisk. Let it boil for 1 to 2 minutes; then remove from the heat. Set aside.

9 Stir the simmering meat and vegetable sauce really well, and remove it from the heat. Add the chia seeds, stirring well to ensure they're dispersed evenly.

10 Bring a large saucepan of water to a boil, and add the ½ teaspoon salt. Add the lasagna, and cook for 5 minutes. Drain the lasagna into a colander and blot dry with paper towels.

11 Preheat the oven to 350 degrees.

12 Spoon one-third of the meat and vegetable sauce into a 9-x-13-inch baking dish. Cover with a layer of 4 lasagna sheets.

13 Spoon one-third of the white sauce over the lasagna sheets and sprinkle 1 tablespoon of cheese over the sauce.

14 Repeat with meat and vegetable sauce, lasagna sheets, white sauce, and cheese until everything is gone. Keep most of the cheese for the top layer.

15 Place the lasagne in the oven and cook for 30 minutes until the cheese on top is golden.

Per serving: Calories 482 (From Fat 233); Fat 26g (Saturated 12g); Cholesterol 96mg; Sodium 707mg; Carbohydrate 32g (Dietary Fiber 4g); Protein 31g.

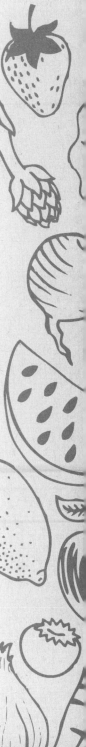

Pasta with Tomato Sauce

Prep time: 15 min • **Cook time:** 20 min • **Yield:** 4 servings

Ingredients	Directions
2 tablespoons olive oil	**1** In a large saucepan, heat the oil over medium heat.
1 medium onion	
2 large carrots	**2** Peel and finely chop the onion; add to the saucepan and cook for 5 minutes.
1 zucchini	
½ cup button mushrooms	**3** Peel and roughly chop the carrots and zucchini; add to the saucepan. Roughly chop the mushrooms; add to the saucepan. Roughly chop the bell pepper; add to the saucepan. Sauté the vegetables for 3 to 4 minutes.
1 red bell pepper	
2 cups dry fusilli or penne pasta	
2 cups passata (see the Note below)	**4** Meanwhile, in a large saucepan of salted water over medium heat, cook the pasta according to the package instructions; set aside.
1 teaspoon soft brown sugar	
1 teaspoon balsamic vinegar	**5** Add the passata, brown sugar, and vinegar to the vegetables and cook everything for another 6 to 8 minutes. Add the vegetable stock; bring to a boil. Simmer everything for another 2 or 3 minutes, stirring occasionally.
3 cups vegetable stock	
2 tablespoons milled chia seeds	
A handful of fresh basil leaves	**6** Remove from the heat and transfer to a blender. Add the milled chia and basil leaves to the blender. Blitz everything on high for a couple minutes or until smooth.
Salt, to taste	
Pepper, to taste	
	7 Drain the cooked pasta, return it to its saucepan, and add the tomato sauce. Stir well before serving.

Per serving: Calories 310 (From Fat 76); Fat 9g (Saturated 1g); Cholesterol 0mg; Sodium 1,060mg; Carbohydrate 53g (Dietary Fiber 7g); Protein 10g.

Note: Passata is blended whole tomatoes, but not reduced to a paste like tomato puree is. You may need to look hard to find it in your local grocery store, but it's typically near the canned tomato products. If you can't find passata in your grocery store, you can use tomato puree instead.

Fish Fingers, Chips, and Beans

Prep time: 15 min • **Cook time:** 30 min • **Yield:** 4 servings

Ingredients	Directions
2 large sweet potatoes	*1* Preheat the oven to 400 degrees.
2 tablespoons olive oil	
1 cup navy beans, drained and rinsed	*2* Cut the sweet potatoes in half widthwise, and then continue cutting lengthwise, until they're in smaller wedges. Pat dry with paper towel and lay on a baking sheet. Drizzle the potatoes with 1 tablespoons of the oil, and toss until coated well. Bake for 20 to 30 minutes, depending on how thick you cut the potatoes.
1 cup passata (see the Note with the preceding recipe)	
1 teaspoon Dijon mustard	
2 tablespoons Worcestershire sauce	*3* While the potatoes are baking, put the beans in a medium saucepan with the passata, mustard, Worcestershire sauce, maple syrup, and tomato puree. Bring to a boil over high heat; turn down the heat and simmer for 20 minutes.
1 tablespoon pure maple syrup	
2 tablespoons tomato puree	
1 pound hoki filets or other firm white fish	*4* Meanwhile, cut the fish into ½-inch strips.
1 cup polenta	*5* On a large plate, mix the polenta, chia, and paprika together; season with salt and pepper.
2 tablespoons milled chia seeds	
2 teaspoons paprika (optional)	*6* In a small bowl, beat the egg. Dip each strip of fish, one at a time, into the egg and then into the polenta mixture until evenly coated. Repeat with all the fish strips.
Salt, to taste	
Pepper, to taste	
1 egg	*7* Add the remaining 1 tablespoon of oil to a separate baking sheet, and lay the fish strips on the baking sheet. Five minutes before the potatoes are ready, add the fish to the oven and bake for 8 minutes, turning halfway through.
	8 Serve the beans alongside the fish strips and sweet potato wedges.

Per serving: Calories 517 (From Fat 95); Fat 11g (Saturated 2g); Cholesterol 108mg; Sodium 885mg; Carbohydrate 70g (Dietary Fiber 11g); Protein 38g.

Chicken Noodle Soup

Prep time: 20 min • **Cook time:** 40 min • **Yield:** 4 servings

Ingredients	Directions
1 tablespoon olive oil	*1* In a large frying pan, heat the olive oil over medium heat.
2 large chicken breasts (approximately 1 pound)	*2* Cut the chicken breasts into thin strips, and add them to the frying pan; cook for 3 to 4 minutes. Add the onion to the pan and cook for another 8 minutes, stirring occasionally to ensure all the chicken cooks through.
1 onion, peeled and thinly sliced	
2 carrots	
1 stick celery	*3* Peel and thinly slice the carrots; add to the pan. Thinly slice the celery stick; add to the pan. Cut the tops and tails off the green beans and chop into very short sticks; add to the pan, mixing everything together and cooking for 5 minutes.
½ cup green beans	
1 garlic clove	
4 cups vegetable stock	
2 sprigs thyme	*4* Peel and mince the garlic clove; add to the pan and cook for another 2 minutes.
1 small bunch parsley	
Salt, to taste	*5* Meanwhile, in a large saucepan, bring the vegetable stock to a boil.
Pepper, to taste	
½ pound thin egg noodles	*6* Tip everything from the frying pan into the vegetable stock and bring to a boil. Add more water if you think it needs it or you prefer a lighter broth.
2 tablespoons whole chia seeds	
	7 Finely chop the thyme and parsley; add to the soup. Season with salt and pepper; simmer for 20 minutes.
	8 In a medium saucepan, bring salted water to a boil and cook the noodles according to the package instructions. Drain and rinse the noodles under cold running water.
	9 Add the noodles and chia seeds to the soup; return to a simmer.

Per serving: Calories 443 (From Fat 91); Fat 10g (Saturated 2g); Cholesterol 137mg; Sodium 1,192mg; Carbohydrate 51g (Dietary Fiber 6g); Protein 35g.

Tip! To make a larger portion to feed more hungry mouths, or if you want the soup to last a couple days, simply double or triple the ingredients.

Keeping Them Going with Snacks

All kids need to snack — their small tummies need to take in food every so often to keep up with their high energy needs. But there's no point providing healthy dinners if you let them snack on potato chips and chocolate all day.

If you've spent any time perusing the snack aisles at your local grocery store, you're probably well aware of all the cheap snacks marketed at kids. Keep healthy snacks on hand for your kids to munch on, and you'll have a better chance of not resorting to the bad stuff. If pester power is just too much for you, try leaving the kids at home next time you shop.

Chia seeds can help you ensure that your children get good nutrition throughout the day. Try the following ways to include chia at kids' snack time:

- **Trail mix:** Add a couple spoons of chia throughout the mix.
- **Yogurt:** Mix chia through their favorite yogurts.
- **Fruit:** Dip cut-up pieces of fresh fruit into a bowl of chia.
- **Cheese:** Add chia to a grilled cheese sandwich.
- **Whole-grain cereal:** Sprinkle chia over healthy cereals.
- **Fruit smoothie:** Add milled chia to the smoothie and blend.

The recipes in this section are great for filling hungry tummies with healthy snacks after school to keep up with kids' energy needs.

Chia Quesadillas

Prep time: 5 min • **Cook time:** 5 min • **Yield:** 2 servings

Ingredients	Directions
2 bacon strips	*1* In a large frying pan, cook the bacon over medium heat until crisp. Drain the bacon on paper towels; set aside to cool.
2 tablespoons cream cheese, softened	
1 tablespoon whole chia seeds	*2* In a small bowl, mix the cream cheese and chia together until the seeds are evenly dispersed.
2 flour tortillas	
1 large tomato	*3* Take a tortilla and spread half of it with the cream cheese mixture.
½ cup grated cheddar cheese	
2 tablespoons plain yogurt	*4* Trim the fat off 1 strip of bacon, and chop the bacon into smaller pieces. Top the cream cheese with the bacon pieces.
Squeezed juice from ½ lime	
2 tablespoons chopped chives	*5* Slice the tomato and place half the slices over the bacon. Top with ¼ cup of the cheese.
Salt, to taste	
Pepper, to taste	*6* Spray a frying pan with cooking oil. Fold the tortilla in half, and place it on the frying pan. Cook each side over low heat for about 1 minute, until the cheese has melted.
	7 Cut the tortilla in 3 wedges.
	8 Repeat with the other tortilla.
	9 In a small bowl, mix the yogurt with the lime juice and the chopped chives. Stir well, and season with salt and pepper.
	10 Serve the dip with the quesadillas.

Per serving: Calories 354 (From Fat 195); Fat 22g (Saturated 11g); Cholesterol 55mg; Sodium 653mg; Carbohydrate 25g (Dietary Fiber 4g); Protein 16g.

Mini Pizzas

Prep time: 5 min • **Cook time:** 10 min • **Yield:** 6 servings

Ingredients	Directions
1 tablespoon olive oil	*1* In a medium frying pan, heat the oil over medium heat.
1 small onion	*2* Chop the onion, add it to the frying pan, and cook for 5 to 6 minutes.
One 15-ounce can chopped tomatoes	
2 tablespoons tomato paste	*3* Add the chopped tomatoes, tomato paste, vegetable stock, brown sugar, vinegar, and oregano, and cook for another 10 minutes.
½ cup vegetable stock	
1 teaspoon soft brown sugar	
1 teaspoon balsamic vinegar	*4* Remove from the heat, and transfer to a blender. Add the milled chia seeds and blend until smooth. Season with salt and pepper.
1 teaspoon dried oregano	
2 tablespoons milled chia seeds	
Salt, to taste	*5* Preheat the broiler to high.
Pepper, to taste	*6* Toast the pitas under the grill for 2 to 3 minutes and remove.
6 small round pitas	
6 cherry tomatoes	*7* Spread the pizza sauce evenly among the 6 pitas and store any remaining sauce covered in the refrigerator for up to three days.
1 red bell pepper	
18 pieces of pepperoni	
¼ cup olives	*8* Cut the cherry tomatoes in half if you're using them for eyes as part of a face. Thinly slice the bell pepper.
1 cup grated mozzarella cheese	
¼ cup sweet corn	*9* Top each pita with a mixture of the tomatoes, bell pepper, pepperoni, olives, cheese, and corn, making faces if you feel like it.
	10 Place under the grill for approximately 4 minutes, until the cheese melts.

Per serving: Calories 236 (From Fat 92); Fat 10g (Saturated 4g); Cholesterol 21mg; Sodium 748mg; Carbohydrate 27g (Dietary Fiber 4g); Protein 10g.

Tip: Kids love to make their own pizzas, and this recipe is perfect for getting them involved in the kitchen!

Vegetable Tempura

Prep time: 10 min • **Cook time:** 10 min • **Yield:** 4 servings

Ingredients	Directions
1 tablespoon sesame seeds	**1** Heat a small frying pan over medium heat; add the sesame seeds. Cook for 3 to 4 minutes, until lightly toasted.
1 tablespoon whole chia seeds	
2 tablespoons smooth peanut butter	**2** In a medium bowl, place the sesame seeds, chia seeds, peanut butter, soy sauce, vinegar, cold water, sugar, and chili powder (if desired). Whisk until well combined and smooth.
1 tablespoon dark soy sauce	
1 tablespoon rice wine vinegar	
1 tablespoon cold water	**3** In a measuring cup, beat the egg yolks with the ice-cold water.
2 teaspoons super-fine sugar	
½ teaspoon chili powder (optional)	**4** In a large bowl, mix the flour and cornstarch; pour the egg mixture into the bowl, and mix together with a fork. The mixture should have a lumpy consistency.
2 egg yolks	
1½ cups ice-cold water	**5** Peel the zucchini and carrots, and cut into sticks.
1½ cups flour	
1 teaspoon cornstarch	**6** Wash the asparagus spears and pat dry with paper towel.
1 zucchini	
2 carrots	**7** Wash and cut the tops and tails off the green beans and pat dry.
6 asparagus spears	
½ cup green beans	**8** Make sure that all the veggies are thoroughly dry.
Sunflower oil for frying	
	9 Fill a saucepan one-third full of the sunflower oil and heat to 350 degrees, using a candy thermometer to check the temperature.
	10 Dip the vegetables in the batter and fry them in batches in the oil for 2 to 3 minutes.
	11 Remove with a slotted spoon and serve with the peanut dipping sauce.

Per serving: Calories 443 (From Fat 199); Fat 22 g (Saturated 3g); Cholesterol 92mg; Sodium 292mg; Carbohydrate 51g (Dietary Fiber 6g); Protein 12g.

Cheesy Chia Potato Skins

Prep time: 15 min • **Cook time:** 1 hr 10 min • **Yield:** 8 servings

Ingredients	*Directions*
2 large baking potatoes	*1* Preheat the oven to 400 degrees.
1 tablespoon olive oil	
4 strips bacon	*2* Scrub the potatoes clean, prick with a fork all over, and brush with the oil. Place in the oven and bake for 40 minutes, until cooked through.
½ teaspoon paprika (optional)	
¼ cup grated cheddar cheese	*3* Cut the bacon into small pieces, and place in a medium frying pan. Cook for 5 to 6 minutes, tossing occasionally, until the bacon is lightly browned.
¼ cup grated mozzarella cheese	
3 scallions, chopped	*4* Cut the potatoes in half, and scoop out the flesh with a spoon, leaving a thin layer of potato so that the skins remain firmly intact. Cut each potato in half again lengthways, to make wedges. Place the potatoes on a baking sheet and sprinkle the paprika over the potatoes (if desired). Top with half the bacon pieces.
2 tablespoons whole chia seeds	
⅓ cup sour cream	
2 tablespoons fresh chives, chopped	*5* In a small bowl, mix the cheddar and mozzarella cheeses, scallions, and chia seeds. Sprinkle the mixture over the potatoes. Top with the remaining pieces of bacon.
	6 Return the potato skins to the oven until golden and crispy.
	7 Meanwhile, in a separate bowl, mix together the sour cream and chives. Serve the dip alongside the potato skins.

Per serving: Calories 119 (From Fat 69); Fat 8g (Saturated 3g); Cholesterol 15mg; Sodium 123mg; Carbohydrate 8g (Dietary Fiber 2g); Protein 5g.

Boosting Kids' Sweet Treats with Chia

What kid doesn't love sweets? As a parent, sometimes you just have to give in and satisfy their cravings — you can't expect them to eat healthy foods all the time. The problem is, commercially manufactured sweet treats are made with cheap, unhealthy ingredients, and laced with sugar, saturated fats, and additives and preservatives that we should all avoid. So, next time you're satisfying your little one's sweet tooth, bake your own sweet treats.

The good news is, baking can be a ton of fun for boys and girls of all ages. They love the messiness of measuring out the ingredients and mixing everything together. As kids get older, they enjoy the challenge of following the recipes and maybe even getting a bit creative themselves. If you can instill a love of baking in your household, chances are, when they're adults themselves, they'll continue to bake family favorites for parties and celebrations — or just an occasional treat.

Chia is a fantastic addition to sweet treats because you can boost the nutrient content without affecting the taste. Often, the texture of baked goods completely hides the seeds, so you can get all those nutrients into your kids without their suspecting a thing.

Chia Fruit Sundae

Prep time: 10 min • **Yield:** 4 servings

Ingredients	Directions
1 cup fresh strawberries	*1* Wash the strawberries and remove the green hulls, and put them in a blender. Blend until the strawberries are completely smooth, with no lumps.
Juice of ½ lemon	
1 tablespoon confectioner's sugar	*2* Pour the strawberry puree through a sieve, pressing it through the sieve with the back of a spoon. Collect the strawberry juice in a bowl.
1 ripe mango	
1 kiwi	*3* Squeeze a little lemon juice into the bowl, and add the confectioner's sugar, stirring well. Set aside.
½ cup fresh raspberries	
½ cup fresh strawberries	*4* Peel and slice the mango, carefully removing the center stone.
8 scoops vanilla ice cream	
2 tablespoons whole chia seeds	*5* Peel the kiwi, and slice it thinly.
2 tablespoons toasted slivered almonds	*6* Wash the raspberries and strawberries and pat dry with paper towel. Cut the berries in half or quarters, depending on the size of the fruit.
	7 Put 1 scoop of vanilla ice cream in the bottom of a tall glass. Add some of the mixed fruit, and sprinkle over some chia seeds. Spoon some strawberry sauce over the fruit and add another scoop of ice cream. Follow with more of the mixed fruit, more chia seeds, and more strawberry sauce. Finish with a scoop of ice cream, and top with the almonds. Repeat with the other 3 glasses.

Per serving: Calories 278 (From Fat 101); Fat 11g (Saturated 5g); Cholesterol 29mg; Sodium 55mg; Carbohydrate 43g (Dietary Fiber 6g); Protein 5g.

Apple and Cinnamon Chia Flapjacks

Prep time: 10 min • **Cook time:** 25 min • **Yield:** 12 servings

Ingredients	Directions
2 Golden Delicious apples	*1* Preheat the oven to 325 degrees.
½ cup butter	
½ cup soft brown sugar	*2* Put some parchment paper under a 8-x-8-inch pan. Draw around the pan with a pencil. Cut out the rectangle of parchment paper. Grease the pan with a little butter, and lay the parchment into the tin.
2 tablespoons pure maple syrup	
½ teaspoon ground cinnamon	
2 tablespoons raisins	*3* Peel the apples, cut them into quarters, remove the cores, and chop them into small chunks. In a medium saucepan, put the chunks of apple with 1 tablespoon of the butter. Cook the apple over low heat for 10 minutes, stirring occasionally until the apple is soft.
3 cups rolled oats	
2 tablespoons whole chia seeds	
	4 Add the rest of the butter to the saucepan along with the brown sugar, maple syrup, cinnamon, and raisins. Heat the mixture gently over low heat until the butter has melted; then remove the pan from the heat. Stir in the oats and chia seeds, combining everything well.
	5 Spoon the mixture into the pan and spread it out, pushing the mixture into the corners with the back of a spoon until it's smooth.
	6 Put the pan in the oven and bake for 25 minutes. The flapjacks should be golden brown and soft when they come out of the oven. They'll get crunchier as they cool. Allow them to cool for 10 minutes before removing from the tray and cutting into squares.

Per serving: Calories 211 (From Fat 87); Fat 10g (Saturated 5g); Cholesterol 20mg; Sodium 5mg; Carbohydrate 30g (Dietary Fiber 3g); Protein 3g.

Mini Baked Raspberry Cheesecakes

Prep time: 15 min • **Cook time:** 25 min • **Yield:** 16 servings

Ingredients	Directions
1 cup graham crackers, broken into pieces **3 tablespoons butter** **2 tablespoons whole chia seeds** **1 cup fresh raspberries** **1 tablespoon icing sugar** **1 pound cream cheese, at room temperature** **¾ cup sugar** **Pinch of salt** **½ teaspoon vanilla extract** **2 eggs**	*1* Preheat the oven to 325 degrees and line a muffin tin with 16 liners. *2* Put the graham crackers into a resealable plastic bag and hit them with a rolling pin until they're well crushed. *3* In a small saucepan, heat the butter over low heat. Remove the saucepan from the heat, and mix the graham crackers and chia seeds into the butter. Spoon 1 tablespoon of the biscuit mixture into each paper liner and press down with the back of a spoon. Bake for about 5 minutes. Remove from the oven and set aside to cool. *4* Meanwhile, in a food processor, blend the raspberries until smooth; strain the fruit through a sieve, pushing the juices through. Discard the raspberry solids. Add the icing sugar to the collected juices, and mix well. Set aside. *5* In a large bowl, whisk the cream cheese using an electric mixer until it's light and fluffy. Gradually add the sugar until it's fully incorporated. Add the raspberry sauce, salt, and vanilla extract. Add the eggs one at a time, beating only until combined after each one, to ensure you don't get too much air into the mixture at this stage. *6* Add 3 tablespoons of the cheesecake filling to each biscuit base in the muffin tin. Return to the oven for 20 minutes or until the cheesecakes are just set. Allow to cool completely in the refrigerator for at least 4 hours before serving.

Per serving: Calories 200 (From Fat 121); Fat 14g (Saturated 7g); Cholesterol 60mg; Sodium 139mg; Carbohydrate 18g (Dietary Fiber 1g); Protein 3g.

Part IV
Boosting Your Baked Goods with Chia

Top Five Quick Chia Snacks

- Spread 1 tablespoon of peanut butter on one slice of whole-grain toast. Top it with half a sliced banana, and sprinkle with 1 tablespoon of whole chia seeds.

- In a bowl, mix ½ cup of oats, ½ cup of mixed nuts, 2 tablespoons of whole chia seeds, and 1 cup of your choice of milk.

- In a blender, blend 1 frozen banana, ½ cup of frozen mixed berries, ½ cup of plain yogurt, 1 cup of orange juice, and 1 tablespoon of milled chia seeds.

- Cut up some carrots, celery sticks, and cucumber into sticks, and dip into your favorite nut butter mixed with 1 tablespoon of milled chia seeds.

- Slice 1 banana, 1 apple, and a handful of strawberries, and mix together in a bowl with ½ cup of Greek yogurt. Sprinkle with 1 tablespoon of whole chia seeds.

Find out how to use chia for endurance in a free article at www.dummies.com/extras/cookingwithchia.

In this part . . .

- ✔ Develop bread recipes full of nutrients.

- ✔ Plan on-the-go snacks to have ready when hunger hits so you aren't tempted to snack on unhealthy foods.

- ✔ Make your everyday lunchbox healthier and more nutritious.

- ✔ Enjoy sweet treats, cakes, and desserts, with the nutrient boost of chia.

Chapter 13

Delicious Breads, Muffins, and Jams

In This Chapter

▶ Making whole-meal, whole-grain, and multi-seed breads

▶ Rising to the occasion with yeast breads

▶ Trying your hand at traditional loaves

▶ Making sweet and savory breads healthier

Bread has been around for over 30,000 years and is a big part of many people's day-to-day food intake. Every country has its own variant of bread, and each in its own way has some basic similar ingredients. Flatbread was said to be the first form of bread; today, many different varieties exist.

Bread is a staple food prepared by baking dough made of flour and water. Salt, fat, and agents such as yeast and baking soda are common ingredients, although bread can contain many other ingredients such as eggs, milk, and sugar.

Chia works well with all varieties of bread. Chia's physical properties means that it can be used as an egg replacement in some recipes. The milled form of chia can also act as flour in some breads. The nutrient profile of chia gives bread a great nutritional boost and is an easy way for people to get chia seeds into their diets.

Whole-Meal, Whole-Wheat, and Multi-Seed Breads

Many people think that bread is fattening, but bread can actually be your friend in a healthy diet. Bread is naturally low in fat and high in fiber. Plus, it's so versatile! You can easily eat many servings a day in place of other high-calorie foods — just don't pile the spreads on your bread.

Whole-wheat bread, in particular, is good for a number of reasons: It's high in complex carbohydrates, low in saturated fat, and brimming with nutrients. Adding seeds like chia to the whole wheat boosts the nutrients.

Growing evidence suggests that replacing refined varieties of grain-based food with whole grains can play a vital role in protecting against disease and improving health. The whole grain contains all three layers of the natural grain, just as nature intended. When the whole grain is refined (like you see in white bread), one or more of the three layers are removed. Only when all three layers are together do you get the health benefits of the whole grain.

People's recommended daily intake of grain-based foods differs greatly depending on age and physical activity but it's a good idea to try to make at least half the grains you eat in a day whole grain. The recipes in this section are some great options.

Multi-seed breads build on the benefits of whole-grain breads by adding seeds to give a super nutritional kick. In addition to the health benefits, seeds work brilliantly in breads and give great flavor and variety to the bread. Chia itself as a whole seed gives a nice crunch in a bread. Adding other seeds like pumpkin, sunflower, and poppy give some fabulous flavors. No matter what bread you make, never be afraid to add seeds, especially chia.

Off the shelf

You may see breads in supermarkets that have very long shelf lives. Manufacturers do this by using preservatives. Be concerned when you see breads on shelves with an unusually long shelf life and try to avoid them. The fresher the bread and the quicker it goes bad, the better it is for you. If you know you won't eat a loaf of bread before it goes bad, simply freeze some of it until you need it. It'll taste just as fresh after you defrost it. Bread will keep in the freezer for 6 months.

Whole-Meal Chia Bread

Prep time: 1 hr • **Cook time:** 30 min • **Yield:** 12 servings

Ingredients	Directions
One ¼-ounce packet active dry yeast	**1** In a small bowl, dissolve the yeast in the lukewarm water; add the brown sugar and malt extract.
1¼ cup lukewarm water	
1 teaspoon brown sugar	**2** In a small saucepan, slightly warm the milk. Add it to the yeast mixture.
¼ tablespoon malt extract	
⅔ cup skim milk	**3** In a large bowl, sift the rye flour, bread flour, and whole-wheat flour; add the oats and 2 teaspoons of the salt.
½ cup rye flour	
1¼ cups bread flour	**4** Make a crater in the center of the flour mixture; pour in the dissolved yeast mixture and the margarine. Knead until a soft dough forms. Add 5 tablespoons of the chia and mix through until well dispersed.
1¼ cups whole-wheat flour	
4 tablespoons rolled oats	
3 teaspoons salt	
4 tablespoons light margarine, softened	**5** Transfer the dough to a lightly greased bowl and cover with plastic wrap. Leave it to stand in a warm place for 1 to 2 hours, until it has doubled in size. Knead the dough again.
5 tablespoons whole chia seeds, plus extra for top of loaf	
1 egg	**6** Preheat the oven to 400 degrees.
¼ cup water	**7** Transfer the dough to a medium loaf pan, cover again with plastic wrap, and let sit for 20 minutes.
1 teaspoon sugar	
	8 Meanwhile, make the browning. In a small bowl, combine the egg, the ¼ cup water, the remaining teaspoon of salt, and the sugar; mix together.
	9 After the dough has sat for 20 minutes, brush it with the browning and sprinkle the loaf with whole chia seeds.
	10 Bake for 30 minutes. Remove from the oven, wrap the bread in a tea towel, and place it on a baking tray to cool.

Per serving: Calories 184 (From Fat 44); Fat 5g (Saturated 1g); Cholesterol 16mg; Sodium 625mg; Carbohydrate 29g (Dietary Fiber 5g); Protein 7g.

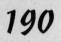

Whole-Wheat Chia Bread

Prep time: 30 min • **Cook time:** 30 min • **Yield:** 16 servings

Ingredients	Directions
1 cup whole-wheat flour	*1* Preheat the oven to 400 degrees. Grease and line two 3½-x-9-inch loaf pans.
2 cups unbleached white flour	
1 teaspoon baking soda	*2* In a large mixing bowl, sift the whole-wheat flour and white flour. Add the baking soda, sugar, and salt.
1 teaspoon sugar	
½ teaspoon sea salt	*3* Add the milled chia seeds, pumpkin seeds, sesame seeds, and sunflower seeds.
⅓ cup milled chia seeds	
⅓ cup pumpkin seeds	*4* Add the buttermilk, and stir to create a soft dough.
¼ cup sesame seeds	
⅓ cup sunflower seeds	*5* Divide the dough in two, and distribute evenly between the loaf pans.
1¾ cups buttermilk	
2 tablespoons whole chia seeds	*6* Sprinkle 1 tablespoon of whole chia seeds over the top of each loaf; press the chia into the loaves.
	7 Bake for 30 to 35 minutes, until the bread is firm in the center.
	8 Wrap the loaves in tea towels and allow them to cool.

Per serving: Calories 155 (From Fat 48); Fat 5g (Saturated 1g); Cholesterol 0mg; Sodium 184mg; Carbohydrate 21g (Dietary Fiber 3g); Protein 6g.

Whole-Wheat French Chia Bread

Prep time: 30 min • **Cook time:** 30 min • **Yield:** 8 servings

Ingredients	*Directions*
1 tablespoon dry yeast	*1* In a small bowl, combine the yeast and the water; sprinkle the sugar over it. Leave for about 5 minutes, until you see the yeast bubbling on top.
1¼ cups lukewarm water	
1 tablespoon sugar	
3 cups whole-wheat flour	*2* In a large bowl, combine the flour, salt, oil, and 1½ tablespoons of the chia. When the yeast is ready, add it to the flour mixture.
½ teaspoon salt	
1½ tablespoons olive oil	*3* Knead the dough by hand for a few minutes until it starts to form a ball. Then pull the dough away from the sides of the bowl and keep the mixture together.
2 tablespoons whole chia seeds	
	4 Cover the bowl with a towel and place it in a warm area; let the dough rise for about 1 hour, until the dough doubles in size.
	5 Preheat the oven to 375 degrees. Grease a baking sheet.
	6 While the oven is heating, roll your dough in a baguette length; place it on the baking sheet. Let it rise again for about 30 minutes and then, with a sharp knife, cut the top of the dough diagonally.
	7 Brush the top of the dough with a little water. Sprinkle the remaining ½ tablespoon of chia onto the dough.
	8 Bake the bread for 30 to 35 minutes or until golden brown. Remove the bread from the pan, wrap it in a towel, and let it cool.

Per serving: Calories 199 (From Fat 41); Fat 5g (Saturated 1g); Cholesterol 0mg; Sodium 145mg; Carbohydrate 36g (Dietary Fiber 6g); Protein 7g.

Multi-Seed Chia Bread

Prep time: 30 min • **Cook time:** 30 min • **Yield:** 12 servings

Ingredients	*Directions*
1½ cups lukewarm water	**1** In a large mixing bowl, combine the water, yeast, and 2½ tablespoons of the honey. Stir to dissolve. Add the bread flour or all-purpose flour; mix. Let this mixture set for 30 minutes. It should be quite loose and not like dough.
2¼ teaspoons active dry yeast	
5 teaspoons honey	
2½ cups bread flour or all-purpose flour	**2** After 30 minutes, mix in 1½ tablespoons of the melted butter, the remaining 2½ tablespoons of honey, and the salt. Mix in the whole and milled chia seeds, sunflower seeds, and wheat germ. Add 1½ cups of the whole-wheat flour.
2½ tablespoons melted butter	
1½ teaspoons salt	
3 tablespoons whole chia seeds	**3** Knead the dough until it's just pulling away from the surface but still sticky to the touch. Add the additional ½ cup of whole wheat flour as needed. Place the dough in a greased bowl. Coat the surface of the dough with the sunflower oil, cover with a damp towel, and let it rise in a warm place until it has doubled in size, about 1 to 1½ hours. Punch down the dough, and shape it into a 15-x-3-inch loaf. Place it in a greased baking dish and make slits in the dough to pattern.
3 tablespoons milled chia seeds	
3 tablespoons sunflower seeds	
3 tablespoons wheat germ	
2 cups whole-wheat flour	**4** Preheat the oven to 350 degrees.
1 tablespoon sunflower oil	
	5 Allow the dough to rise by about an inch. Bake the dough for 30 to 35 minutes. Keep an eye on it and be sure not to overbake. When the bread is done baking, remove it from the oven and lightly brush the top with the remaining 1 tablespoon of melted butter to prevent the top from crusting too hard.

Per serving: Calories 252 (From Fat 62); Fat 7g (Saturated 2g); Cholesterol 6mg; Sodium 293mg; Carbohydrate 41g (Dietary Fiber 5g); Protein 8g.

Yeast Breads

Yeast is a live organism that feeds on sugar and moisture to live and reproduce. Yeast itself has been identified as one of the earliest domesticated organisms and has been used in the baking process for fermentation throughout history. It has many other uses through the fermentation of sugars, and many variations of yeast are used for the baking process. Yeast is also used in the production of beer, wine, nonalcoholic beverages, and nutritional supplements, to name a few.

Here are some tips for working with yeast:

✔ When in a good state, yeast has a light gray color and a distinctive aroma.

✔ The standard proportion of fresh yeast for bread making is 1¾ ounces to every 2 pounds of flour. If you use too much yeast, the bread becomes sharp and turns stale quickly. If you follow the recipes in this book, you'll be fine.

✔ The liquid used when yeast is dissolved must be lukewarm. If you have the temperature too high, it will kill the ferment.

✔ The ideal temperature for leavening is 75 to 85 degrees.

✔ You can tell that dough has leavened enough by placing a small amount of the dough into water — if it floats, the leavening is good.

✔ Never substitute baking powder for yeast.

Chia and Lemon Pull-Apart Bread

Prep time: 1 hr 15 min • **Cook time:** 30 min • **Yield:** 12 servings

Ingredients	Directions
¼ cup lukewarm water	**1** In a small bowl, place the water, yeast, and 1 teaspoon out of the ¼ cup of sugar. Allow to sit for 5 minutes, until it foams or bubbles.
One ¼-ounce packet dry active yeast	
1¼ cups sugar (separated into 1 cup and ¼ cup)	**2** In a large bowl, combine the flour, the remainder of the ¼ cup of sugar, the salt, and the chia; stir together.
3 cups flour	**3** In a small saucepan over low heat, melt 4 tablespoons of the butter with the milk, until it's just melted; remove from the heat.
½ teaspoon salt	
¼ cup whole chia seeds	**4** Pour the yeast mixture into the flour; then pour the milk into the flour, and stir. Add the eggs and vanilla extract, and stir. Use your hands to knead the dough into a ball. Place the dough in a lightly greased bowl, cover, and let rise for 1 hour.
7 tablespoons butter	
⅓ cup milk	
2 large eggs	**5** While the dough is rising, press the lemon zest in a cup with the remaining 1 cup of sugar to release the oils.
½ teaspoon vanilla extract	
2 teaspoons lemon zest	**6** When the dough is ready, place it on a lightly floured surface, and punch it down and roll it out until it's about ¼ inch thick.
	7 Preheat the oven to 350 degrees.
	8 In a small saucepan, melt the remaining 3 tablespoons of butter and spread over the dough; sprinkle the lemon sugar over the dough evenly.
	9 Cut the dough into long strips. Place the strips over each other and then cut into squares. Place the squares in a lightly greased bread pan. Bake for 30 to 35 minutes. Make sure the top is golden brown and the center isn't raw. Cool before removing from the pan.

Per serving: Calories 289 (From Fat 81); Fat 9g (Saturated 5g); Cholesterol 49mg; Sodium 114mg; Carbohydrate 47g (Dietary Fiber 2g); Protein 5g.

Chia and Walnut Bread

Prep time: 3 hr • **Cook time:** 45 min • **Yield:** 16 servings

Ingredients	Directions
4¾ teaspoons active dry yeast	*1* In a small bowl, dissolve the yeast in ½ cup of the lukewarm water; add the sugar. Let sit for about 5 minutes, until it foams or bubbles.
1½ cups lukewarm water	
1 teaspoon sugar	
3½ cups bread flour	*2* In a large bowl, sift the bread flour, whole-wheat flour, and salt; add the milled chia seeds and whole chia seeds and mix. Create a center in the middle of the mix.
¾ cup whole-wheat flour	
2 teaspoons salt	
4 tablespoons milled chia seeds	*3* Pour the yeast and the remaining 1 cup of lukewarm water into the center of the mix.
1 teaspoons whole chia seeds	*4* Cover with the flour and combine. Knead to obtain a soft dough; add the walnuts and knead again to combine the walnuts well.
¾ cup walnuts, chopped	
	5 Place the dough in a bowl and cover with plastic; leave to stand in a warm area until it doubles in size, about 2 hours.
	6 After the dough has risen, place it on a baking sheet; shape it as you wish, cover it with a tea towel, and leave for 1 hour.
	7 Preheat the oven to 350 degrees. and bake for 45 minutes or until brown and the center sounds hollow.

Per serving: Calories 158 (From Fat 42); Fat 5g (Saturated 1g); Cholesterol 0mg; Sodium 292mg; Carbohydrate 24g (Dietary Fiber 2g); Protein 5g.

Tip: To optimize walnuts' nutrition and storage, buy whole nuts and crack them at the point of using them. If you opt for the more convenient pre-peeled walnuts, keep them in a dry airtight container away from daylight.

Traditional Loaves

The amazing think about bread is its variety. What someone in Ireland thinks is traditional differs from what someone in the United States or Japan thinks is traditional. Tradition is what defines each region. The ingredients and methods used to produce bread in a particular area are handed down from generation to generation. Cultures may have evolved and the ability to cook has gotten easier, but the loaves we eat today have been a part of tradition for generations.

Flatbread is a common type of bread that is used in the traditional loaves of many countries. It's a simple bread made with flour, water, and salt; rolled out; and flattened. Many flatbreads are unleavened and made without yeast, but adding yeast gives a slight leaven, like pita bread. Flatbreads have many other ingredients, depending on the region. They can contain curry powder, chili powder, or black pepper; different flavored oils may be added as well. Flatbreads can range from a few millimeters to a few centimeters thick. Naan bread is a very common flatbread and is native to the regions of Iran, northern India, Pakistan, and Afghanistan. Crisp bread is very common in Scandinavia. China has bread called *bing* that is approximately ¾ inch thick. And tortillas are a very well-known flatbread, native to Mexico.

Leavened types of bread are also common. Leavening is the process of adding gas to the dough through baking soda, self-rising flour, or yeast. Quick bread is native to North America, rye is found in Northern Europe, and zwieback is from Germany.

Some of the other traditional types of bread are yeast, sweet, soda, and sour-dough. Then there are many types that are a mixture, like a leavened flatbread such as pizza.

Chia Flatbread

Prep time: 1 hr 20 min • **Cook time:** 15 min • **Yield:** 6 servings

Ingredients	Directions
1 cup whole-wheat flour 1 cup durum flour ½ teaspoon salt 1 teaspoon instant yeast 2 tablespoons milled chia seeds 2 tablespoons toasted chia seeds 2 tablespoons soft butter ¾ cup lukewarm water 6 teaspoons oil	*1* In a medium bowl, sift the whole-wheat flour and durum flour; add the salt, yeast, milled chia seeds, and toasted chia seeds. Work in the soft butter, and add the water. Mix and knead the dough until it becomes smooth.
	2 Form the dough into a ball and place in a bowl. Cover the bowl with plastic wrap, and place in a warm place for about 1 hour. The dough should get puffy.
	3 Transfer the dough onto a greased surface and fold it several times. Divide it into six pieces; roll each piece into a ball. Cover the dough balls with a damp cloth, and let rest for about 10 minutes. Roll each dough ball into a flat circle, approximately ⅛ inch thick. Use a little extra flour if it gets too sticky.
	4 Heat a frying pan over medium heat; add 1 teaspoon of the oil to the pan just before placing the dough in the pan. Place the first piece of dough in the pan, cook for 1 or 2 minutes, until it starts to bubble and has some darkish brown spots; flip it over and bake the second side until firm.
	5 Continue with each of the remaining pieces of dough, putting a teaspoon of oil in the pan with each, until all the pieces have been cooked.
	6 Stack the flatbreads together on a plate and cover with a clean tea towel to keep them warm. Use within a day to ensure freshness.

Per serving: Calories 281 (From Fat 102); Fat 12g (Saturated 3g); Cholesterol 10mg; Sodium 197mg; Carbohydrate 40g (Dietary Fiber 8g); Protein 8g.

Chia Brown Soda Bread

Prep time: 1 hr 20 min • **Cook time:** 15 min • **Yield:** 6 servings

Ingredients	Directions
2¼ cups whole-wheat flour	**1** Preheat the oven to 350 degrees.
½ cup all-purpose flour	
¼ cup milled chia seeds	**2** In a large bowl, sift the whole-wheat flour and all-purpose flour. Add the milled chia seeds and the oats; combine.
½ cup rolled oats	
2 tablespoons brown sugar	**3** Add the brown sugar, wheat germ, baking soda, baking powder, and salt to the mixture; combine.
1 tablespoon wheat germ	
1 teaspoon baking soda	**4** In a small bowl, slightly beat the egg; add the buttermilk.
1 teaspoon baking powder	
½ teaspoon salt	**5** Create a well in the flour mixture, and pour the egg and buttermilk mixture into the well.
1 egg	
2 cups low-fat buttermilk	**6** Mix the dry and wet ingredients, ensuring that all ingredients are well combined.
3 teaspoons whole chia seeds	
	7 Coat a loaf pan with cooking spray, and pour the mixture into the pan. Scatter the whole chia seeds evenly on top of the mixture.
	8 Bake for approximately 1 hour, until the bread is brown and a knife sliced through the bread comes out dry.
	9 Remove from the oven, let cool slightly, and remove from the pan. Wrap the bread in a tea towel until cool.

Per serving: Calories 311 (From Fat 46); Fat 5g (Saturated 1g); Cholesterol 34mg; Sodium 571mg; Carbohydrate 56g (Dietary Fiber 8g); Protein 13g.

English Muffins and Jam

English muffins are a real treat on a cold day. They're simple to make, but they take a little time because they have to rise to become all lovely and bubbly. The good news: You can make them in advance — they store well for up to two days in an airtight container. English muffins are traditionally served hot, split horizontally, and buttered, but the options are endless. Scrambled eggs and bacon are a fantastic combination with English muffins, but so is chicken and avocado or even peanut butter and blueberries. What you do with English muffins is entirely up to you! You can make them as healthy as you like depending on the toppings you choose.

In this section, we give you a delicious recipe for classic English muffins that are healthier than your average ones thanks to the addition of chia.

These English muffins are still very much a treat and should be consumed in moderation, especially if you like to load them with not-so-healthy toppings.

At the end of this section, we give you two recipes for chia jam. These jams taste just as good as (we think even better than) the traditional kind, but because they contain chia — you guessed it! — they're better for you.

One of our jam recipes uses stevia as an alternative sweetener — this recipe is tasty because the natural sugar of the strawberry boosts the sweetness of the jam.

Both recipes can be made with whatever fruit you like in your jam. Chia acts as the gelling agent to give the jam the consistency you're used to with jam without going through the whole jamming process.

English Muffins with Chia

Prep time: 1½ hr • **Cook time:** 8 min • **Yield:** 12 servings

Ingredients	Directions
1¾ teaspoons dry active yeast 1 cup skim milk, at room temperature 1 teaspoon sugar 5⅔ cups bread flour 1 teaspoon salt 1 egg 5 tablespoons milled chia seeds 3 tablespoons sunflower oil	**1** In a small bowl, place the yeast, milk, and sugar; let sit for 5 minutes, until it bubbles or foams. **2** In a large bowl, mix the flour and salt. **3** In a separate small bowl, lightly beat the egg. **4** Make a well in the center of the flour mixture; pour in the yeast and egg. Mix gently, ensuring that all the ingredients are well combined. After a dough has formed, transfer it to a work table and knead it to obtain a uniform mixture. Transfer the dough to a bowl, cover the bowl with plastic wrap, and leave the dough in a warm place until it doubles in size, about 1 hour. **5** Add the milled chia seeds to the dough and knead again to thoroughly combine. Place the dough in a lightly greased bowl, cover it with a clean tea towel, and allow it to rise again for about 30 minutes. **6** Remove the dough and roll it out until it's about 1 inch thick. Using a 3-inch round cookie cutter, cut out 12 rounds, rerolling the dough if it starts to get puffy and to incorporate any scraps. Place these rounds on a lightly floured baking tray and allow them to rise again for 20 to 25 minutes. **7** In a skillet, heat 1 tablespoon of the sunflower oil. Cook the muffins over low heat for around 6 or 7 minutes per side. You'll probably get 2 or 3 muffins into the skillet at a time, so you'll have to cook them in batches. **8** Repeat with the remaining muffins, adding oil to the skillet as needed.

Per serving: Calories 292 (From Fat 51); Fat 6g (Saturated 1g); Cholesterol 0mg; Sodium 210mg; Carbohydrate 50g (Dietary Fiber 3g); Protein 10g.

Chia Raspberry Jam

Prep time: 15 min • **Cook time:** 10 min • **Yield:** 25 servings

Ingredients	Directions
2 cups drained canned or frozen raspberries	*1* Using a blender, puree the raspberries.
1 cup sugar	*2* Push the pureed fruit through a fine mesh sieve, making sure to collect the juices and discard the seeds that are left in the sieve.
5 tablespoons whole chia seeds	
7 tablespoons water	*3* In a medium bowl, place the sugar and the collected fruit puree (without the seeds). Place the bowl in the refrigerator for 1 hour to allow the sugar to dissolve
	4 Remove from the refrigerator. Add the chia seeds and water.
	5 In a medium saucepan, cook the mixture over a very low heat, stirring occasionally. When the desired jam consistency is obtained, remove from the stove and transfer to a jam jar.

Per serving: Calories 45 (From Fat 6); Fat 1g (Saturated 0g); Cholesterol 0mg; Sodium 0mg; Carbohydrate 10g (Dietary Fiber 1g); Protein 0g.

Chia Strawberry Jam

Prep time: 25 min • **Yield:** 10 servings

Ingredients	Directions
1 cup strawberries	**1** In a medium bowl, mash the strawberries with a fork. If you prefer, place them in a blender and blend them; then transfer to a medium bowl.
1 tablespoon whole chia seeds	
1 tablespoon water	**2** Mix in the chia seeds, water, and stevia.
1 tablespoon stevia, or to taste	
	3 Cover the bowl with plastic, and refrigerate for 20 minutes to set.

Per serving: Calories 10 (From Fat 3); Fat 0g (Saturated 0g); Cholesterol 0mg; Sodium 0mg; Carbohydrate 2g (Dietary Fiber 1g); Protein 0g.

Chapter 14

Chia on the Go

*T*hroughout this book, we show you the many ways that chia can be used, from getting it into your breakfast bowl to boosting your dinner and everything in between. Chia is a highly versatile seed, brimming with nutrients. It can be added to almost everything to boost the nutritional value of your meals.

In today's hectic lifestyle, we sometimes forget to eat properly. It's not that we don't *intend* to eat well — we're just not prepared when we have to rush from work to the gym, to collect the kids at school, and back again. At the grocery store, we're drawn to addictive snack bars and other quick snacks full of sugar and saturated fat. Many of these snacks are mass produced with cheap ingredients devoid of nutrients. But because we're in a rush, we end up buying foods that don't exactly meet our nutritional needs.

With a little preparation, you can make wonderfully nutritious snacks at home that you can store, grab, and eat on the go, while running out the door to wherever life is taking you next. In this chapter, we show you how to create energy bars, trail mixes, and other lunchbox favorites that are full of nutrients our bodies need.

Energy Bars and Trail Mixes

Energy bars are everywhere these days. Go to any health food store or supermarket and you'll find a huge range of energy bars promising to fill you up and give you energy when you need it. These energy bars cater to today's busy lifestyle — people are out and about and need something they can pop into their cars or bags and eat whenever they get hungry.

Energy bars and trail mixes are great, but we recommend making your own and staying away from the often over-processed bars available at your local market. In this section, we give you recipes for snacks that you can make ahead of time and used when you want. They're packed full of nutritious ingredients that are naturally high in good fats, fiber, protein, and antioxidants, but we don't add any refined sugars, preservatives, or other ingredients you don't recognize. By making your own energy bars and trail mixes, you know exactly what you're eating and you can fuel your body with what it needs, conveniently.

Choosing store-bought energy bars

Even though we provide recipes for chia-powered bars you can make at home, you may still find yourself needing to pick something up when you're out and about. If you're reaching for an energy bar at a convenience store, pay attention to the following:

✔ **The ingredient list:** The fewer ingredients on that list, the better. If you don't recognize ingredients on the list, choose a different bar.

✔ **Carbohydrates:** If you're looking for a bar that will give you fuel for your workout, choose a bar that has 40 g or more of carbohydrates. The key is to make sure that only a small amount of these carbs are sugars, so opt for a bar where less than half of its carbs are sugars.

✔ **Fat:** We all need fat in our diets, especially if we're working out, but it's the *kind* of fat that can be worrisome. Choose a different bar if the one you're looking at has more than 1 g or 2 g of saturated fat.

Chia Chocolate Energy Bar

Prep time: 15 min • **Yield:** 12 servings

Ingredients	Directions
1½ cups dates, pitted	*1* In a food processor, puree the dates with the water to form a thick paste.
1 tablespoon water	
⅓ cup dried cranberries	*2* Add the cranberries to the food processor and pulse again.
½ cup whole chia seeds	
⅓ cup cocoa powder	*3* Add the chia seeds, cocoa powder, coconut, vanilla extract, and salt to the food processor. Pulse all the ingredients together until they're well mixed.
⅓ cup unsweetened coconut flakes	
1 teaspoon vanilla extract	
¼ teaspoon sea salt	*4* Transfer the mixture to a large bowl.
¼ cup dark chocolate, chopped	*5* Mix in the dark chocolate, oats, and walnuts.
⅓ cup oats	
1 cup walnut pieces	*6* Cut out a large piece of wax paper to fit an 8-x-8-inch pan, with extra to wrap around the mixture. Line the pan with the wax paper.
	7 Place the mixture into the pan, and press it down into all four corners.
	8 When the mixture is evenly spread in the pan, cover with the remaining wax paper.
	9 Place the pan in the refrigerator and leave overnight.
	10 The next morning, unwrap the mixture and cut it into even bars.
	11 Wrap the bars individually. Keep them in an airtight container in the fridge.

Per serving: Calories 209 (From Fat 99); Fat 11g (Saturated 3g); Cholesterol 0mg; Sodium 52mg; Carbohydrate 28g (Dietary Fiber 6g); Protein 4g.

Superfood Energy Bar

Prep time: 10 min • **Cook time:** 30 min • **Yield:** 12 servings

Ingredients	Directions
1 cup quinoa	**1** Preheat the oven to 375 degrees. Line an 8-x-12-inch pan with wax paper. Fill a medium saucepan with water and bring to a boil.
4 tablespoons whole chia seeds	
1 cup frozen blueberries	**2** Rinse the quinoa in cold water, add it to the boiling water, and let it simmer for approximately 15 minutes. Drain the quinoa, and set it aside to cool. If you have time, let it cool in the refrigerator overnight.
24 dates, pitted	
1 teaspoon vanilla extract	
¼ cup chopped almonds	**3** In a blender, add the chia seeds, blueberries, and dates and blend until it's nice and gooey. Add the vanilla extract and blend again for another 30 seconds.
⅔ cup dried goji berries	
4 ounces dark chocolate, roughly chopped	
	4 In a medium bowl, mix the cooked quinoa, the date mixture, the almonds, and most of the goji berries. Spread the mixture in the lined pan. The consistency will be quiet dense. Bake for around 30 minutes, until crispy. Remove from the oven.
	5 In a small plastic bowl, place the chocolate pieces. Put the bowl over a small saucepan of gently simmering water to melt the chocolate. Cover the date mixture with the melted chocolate.
	6 Chop up the remaining dried goji berries and sprinkle over the chocolate before it sets. Let it cool, cut into portions, and then place in the refrigerator overnight.

Per serving: Calories 182 (From Fat 62); Fat 7g (Saturated 2g); Cholesterol 0mg; Sodium 32mg; Carbohydrate 26g (Dietary Fiber 7g); Protein 5g.

Roasted Nut and Seed Trail Mix

Prep time: 10 min • **Cook time:** 15–20 min • **Yield:** 24 servings

Ingredients	Directions
¼ cup pumpkin seeds	**1** Preheat the oven to 350 degrees.
¼ cup hemp seeds	
¼ cup sunflower seeds	**2** In a dry frying pan, combine the pumpkin seeds, hemp seeds, and sunflower seeds and toast over medium heat, shaking the pan to prevent burning. Stop when the seeds begin to pop.
2 tablespoons coconut oil	
½ cup almonds	
½ cup cashews	**3** Coat a large baking sheet with the coconut oil. Add the almonds, cashews, peanuts, pistachios, hazelnuts, pecans, and pine nuts to the baking sheet. Roast in the oven for 5 minutes. Remove from the oven and stir well, making sure all the nuts make it to the center of the baking tray at some point. Roast for another 3 minutes and take another look. The nuts should roast in a total of 8 to 12 minutes, so be sure to keep an eye on the oven to ensure they don't burn. When the nuts are nicely browned and smell nutty, remove the pan from the oven and allow the nuts to cool; set aside.
½ cup peanuts	
½ cup pistachios	
½ cup hazelnuts	
½ cup pecans	
¼ cup pine nuts	
¼ cup chopped dried apricots	
¼ cup raisins	
¼ cup dried pineapple chunks	**4** In a large bowl, mix the toasted seeds, roasted nuts, apricots, raisins, pineapple, banana chips, chia, and coconut. Sprinkle the ginger, cinnamon, and salt over the mixture, and combine well.
¼ cup banana chips	
½ cup whole chia seeds	
¼ cup desiccated coconut	**5** Store the mixture in a large airtight container.
¼ teaspoon ground ginger	
¼ teaspoon ground cinnamon	
¼ teaspoon salt	

Per serving: Calories 179 (From Fat 129); Fat 14g (Saturated 3g); Cholesterol 0mg; Sodium 29mg; Carbohydrate 10g (Dietary Fiber 3g); Protein 5g.

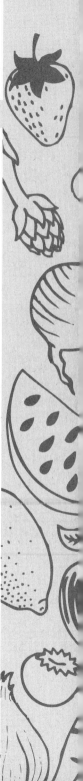

Lunchbox Favorites

Lunchboxes can get so boring, whether you're packing them for kids or yourself. You can easily fall into the habit of making the same sandwiches over and over, and not giving your body the fuel it needs to keep you working at your best. That's where chia can help. By simply adding chia to your favorite lunches, you can load up on omega-3 fatty acids to help with concentration. Plus, the slow-releasing energy will help prevent the slump in the middle of the day that often strikes when you haven't had a good lunch.

You can add chia to anything you already enjoy, so if you're getting tired of packing the same lunch but you're stumped for ideas, get some inspiration from the following list. Just bring some chia seeds packed in a small canister and sprinkle them over any of the following:

- Green leafy salads
- Leftovers
- Soups
- Pasta salads
- Salad wraps
- Quesadillas
- Nachos
- Sandwiches

Cold Pasta and Chia Salad

Prep time: 10 min • **Cook time:** 8–12 min • **Yield:** 3 servings

Ingredients	Directions
¼ teaspoon salt	**1** Fill a medium saucepan with water and bring to a boil; add the salt.
2 cups fusilli or bowtie pasta	
3 scallions, finely sliced	**2** Cook the pasta according to the package instructions, typically 8 to 10 minutes.
1 cup broccoli florets, chopped	
1 cup cherry tomatoes, halved	**3** Drain the pasta into a colander and run cold water over it to help it cool faster; allow it to dry thoroughly.
1 stalk celery, finely sliced	
¼ cucumber, finely sliced	
¼ cup olives	**4** In a large bowl, mix the scallions, broccoli florets, tomatoes, celery, and cucumber.
¼ cup hazelnuts	
2 tablespoons whole chia seeds	**5** Add the olives, hazelnuts, chia, and feta to the bowl, and mix well.
½ cup feta cheese, crumbled	
3 tablespoons extra-virgin olive oil	**6** When the pasta is dry, add it to the salad vegetables and mix well.
1 tablespoon balsamic vinegar	
Sea salt, to taste	**7** In a small jar, put the olive oil, vinegar, sea salt, and pepper. Tighten the lid and shake until well mixed.
Pepper, to taste	
	8 Pour this dressing over the salad, and mix again.

Per serving: Calories 550 (From Fat 281); Fat 32g (Saturated 7g); Cholesterol 0mg; Sodium 865mg; Carbohydrate 55g (Dietary Fiber 7g); Protein 16g.

Tip: If you find the chia seeds to be a little soft when you go to eat your salad and you'd prefer them to be crunchy, simply put the chia seeds into a small resealable bag and bring it with you. You can add the chia seeds to your salad just before you eat it.

Pesto Chicken Sandwich

Prep time: 10 min • **Yield:** 1 serving

Ingredients	Directions
⅓ **cup cooked shredded chicken**	**1** In a small bowl, mix the chicken, pesto, mayonnaise, and chia; stir well to combine.
1 tablespoon basil pesto	
1 tablespoon light mayonnaise	**2** Season with the salt and pepper and spoon the mixture onto a slice of rye bread.
1 tablespoon whole chia seeds	**3** Spread the tomato evenly over the chicken pesto mix, and top with the lettuce.
Salt, to taste	
Pepper, to taste	**4** Close the sandwich with the other slice of rye bread.
2 slices rye bread	
1 tomato, finely sliced	
1 small handful of iceberg lettuce, washed	

Per serving: Calories 437 (From Fat 187); Fat 21g (Saturated 4g); Cholesterol 49mg; Sodium 791mg; Carbohydrate 41g (Dietary Fiber 9g); Protein 22g.

Sandwich options

If you find yourself packing the same sandwiches every day and you're longing for a change, try your hand at the following sandwich options, on your favorite bread:

✔ Roasted turkey breast, cheddar cheese, tomato relish, and arugula

✔ Bacon, brie cheese, apple slices, and pickle

✔ Cooked ham, cream cheese, sliced tomato, and mustard

✔ Roasted mixed peppers, shredded lettuce, and sliced avocado

✔ Roasted chicken, onion stuffing, and cream cheese

✔ Cheddar cheese, cucumber, and thinly sliced red onion

Don't forget the chia! Bring some whole chia seeds with you in a small canister and sprinkle them into your sandwich at lunchtime to give you the energy you need for the rest of the day.

Classic Peanut Butter and Jelly Sandwich

Prep time: 2 min • **Yield:** 1 serving

Ingredients	Directions
2 slices whole-grain bread	*1* Coat one slice of bread with the peanut butter and the other slice of bread with the jelly.
1 tablespoon crunchy peanut butter	
1 tablespoon raspberry jelly	*2* Sprinkle the chia seeds on top of the peanut butter, and place the jelly-coated bread on top, jelly side down.
1 tablespoon whole chia seeds	

Per serving: Calories 333 (From Fat 121); Fat 13g (Saturated 2g); Cholesterol 0mg; Sodium 278mg; Carbohydrate 43g (Dietary Fiber 9g); Protein 13g.

Tuna Mayonnaise Wrap

Prep time: 10 min • **Yield:** 1 serving

Ingredients	Directions
One 3-ounce pouch of tuna in water	*1* In a small bowl, mix the tuna with the mayonnaise, corn, and chia seeds; season with salt and pepper.
1 tablespoon light mayonnaise	
1 teaspoon canned corn	*2* Spread the mixture in the center of the tortilla, top with the lettuce, and roll up.
1 tablespoon whole chia seeds	
Salt, to taste	
Pepper, to taste	
1 whole-wheat tortilla	
½ cup chopped iceberg lettuce	

Per serving: Calories 244 (From Fat 106); Fat 12g (Saturated 2g); Cholesterol 5mg; Sodium 599mg; Carbohydrate 30g (Dietary Fiber 7g); Protein 6g.

Chapter 15

Have Your Cake and Eat It, Too: Chia Desserts

In This Chapter

▶ Baking cupcakes with chia

▶ Making muffins to make your mouth water

▶ Boosting the nutritional profile of your grandmother's cake recipes

▶ Making more sweet treats that everyone loves

*W*ho doesn't love dessert? That sweet treat after a lovely meal is often the best part. Given how much we talk about healthy eating in this book, a chapter on desserts may come as a surprise. But we're big believers in that old adage "Everything in moderation." As long as you don't make the recipes in this chapter part of your daily diet and you keep them for what they were intended for — special treats — you can maintain a healthy diet.

Cupcake Heaven

Cupcakes have grown in popularity recently. Entire shops dedicated to cupcakes are opening all over the United States. And in Beverly Hills, you can even find a "Cupcake ATM" (from Sprinkles Cupcakes). These delicious little single-portion treats are perfect for celebrations. And when you make the effort to decorate them, cupcakes can look as good as they taste.

However, cupcakes do come at a price. The typical cupcake is made from white flour, sugar, butter, and eggs. When you add the buttercream icing that's often piled high on top, you're talking numerous calories and loads of saturated fat. The good news is that the recipes in this section add chia seeds to the mix, which means that your favorite treat will have a nutrient boost.

Lemon and Chia Cupcakes

Prep time: 10 min • **Cook time:** 15 min • **Yield:** 12 servings

Ingredients	Directions
½ cup butter, at room temperature	**1** Preheat the oven to 350 degrees and line a muffin tin with 12 liners.
¼ cup super-fine sugar	
2 eggs	**2** In a large bowl, beat the butter and sugar until the mixture is pale and creamy.
1 teaspoon vanilla extract	
Juice and zest of 1 lemon	**3** Add the eggs one at a time to the mixture, beating the first egg into the mixture before adding the second.
2 cups flour	
1 teaspoon baking powder	**4** Add the vanilla extract, and continue beating.
½ cup 2 percent milk	**5** Add the lemon juice and lemon zest, and beat for about 30 seconds.
3 tablespoons whole chia seeds	
	6 In a separate bowl, sift the flour and baking powder.
	7 Mix the dry ingredients into the wet ingredients.
	8 Add the milk and chia seeds to the mixture, and continue mixing until everything is well combined.
	9 Pour the mixture into the muffin tin.
	10 Bake for 15 minutes.

Per serving: Calories 191 (From Fat 86); Fat 10g (Saturated 5g); Cholesterol 52mg; Sodium 52mg; Carbohydrate 22g (Dietary Fiber 2g); Protein 4g.

Tip: If you want to frost the cupcakes, you can make a simple frosting with 1 cup powdered sugar, 2 tablespoons milk, and ½ teaspoon vanilla extract.

Vary It! The majority of this mixture can make any cupcake. To change the flavor, just change the juice of the fruit you're using.

Vanilla and Chia Buttercream Cupcakes

Prep time: 10 min • **Cook time:** 15–18 min • **Yield:** 16 servings

Ingredients	Directions
1¾ cups butter, at room temperature	**1** Preheat the oven to 350 degrees and line a muffin tin with 16 liners.
1½ cups sugar	
3 eggs	**2** In a large bowl, beat ¾ cup of the butter with an electric mixer for 1 minute, until soft and creamy. Add in the sugar and beat until combined. Add in the eggs and 3 teaspoons of the vanilla extract, and continue to beat for another 1 minute.
3½ teaspoons vanilla extract	
½ teaspoon salt	
2 teaspoons baking powder	
2 cups flour	**3** In a separate bowl, stir together the salt, baking powder, flour, and milled chia seeds.
½ cup milled chia seeds	
1¾ cups 2 percent milk	**4** Gradually add the dry ingredients and the milk to the beaten butter and sugar and mix until well combined. Pour the mixture into the muffin tin.
3 cups powdered sugar	
4 tablespoons heavy whipping cream	**5** Bake for 15 to 18 minutes, or until golden brown and a toothpick comes out clean when inserted into the middle. Allow to cool for at least 30 minutes before frosting.
	6 In another large bowl, beat the remaining 1 cup of butter and the powdered sugar until light and fluffy. Add the remaining ½ teaspoon of vanilla extract, and stir until smooth. Add a little of the heavy whipping cream at a time, until the desired consistency is reached. Put the frosting into a piping bag. Pipe the frosting onto each of the cooled cupcakes.

Per serving: Calories 453 (From Fat 213); Fat 24g (Saturated 14g); Cholesterol 96mg; Sodium 154mg; Carbohydrate 56g (Dietary Fiber 2g); Protein 5g.

Muffin Madness

Muffins can be made to be a lot healthier than cupcakes by adding vegetables such as carrots or zucchini. Plus, you don't normally see muffins piled high with sugary frosting. Nuts and seeds, including chia seeds, are a great addition to muffins. You can also improve the nutrient profile of your muffins by opting for reduced-fat dairy products, trans-fat-free margarine instead of butter, and stevia instead of sugar.

Muffins are often sold in very big portions when you buy them at a bakery or coffee shop, but when you make them at home, you can make them smaller and keep the calorie count down.

Baking tips

The success of any recipe is in the preparation. Here are some quick baking tips. Follow these suggestions, and you're sure to end up with delicious baked goods every time:

✔ Get all the ingredients out and ready to use before you start. Do this early enough so that you allow the ingredients time to come to room temperature (as opposed to using them straight out of the fridge). If you forget to get your eggs out of the refrigerator a few hours before you're ready to start, you can warm them up by placing them in a bowl of warm water. Just get some warm water straight from the tap — no need to heat it on the stove.

✔ Always preheat the oven and line or grease your baking pans, as indicated in the recipe.

✔ As with any recipe, add all the ingredients in the order indicated in the recipe. Don't add a new ingredient until the previous ones have been integrated well into the mixture.

✔ Always sift dry ingredients. And when adding dry ingredients, don't beat the mixture. Instead, fold them in gradually.

✔ When placing the mixture in the oven, put it in the middle of the middle rack.

✔ No matter how tempted you may be, don't open the door during the first half of the baking process.

Chia and Coffee Muffins

Prep time: 15 min • **Cook time:** 15 min • **Yield:** 14 servings

Ingredients	Directions
2 egg whites	*1* Preheat the oven to 350 degrees and line a muffin tin with 14 liners.
1 egg yolk	
⅔ cup unrefined sugar	*2* In a medium bowl, beat the egg whites, egg yolk, and sugar until creamy.
4½ tablespoons sunflower oil	
1 teaspoon vanilla extract	*3* Slowly add the oil while continuing to beat.
2 ounces lowfat cream cheese	
1¾ cups flour	*4* Slowly add the vanilla extract while continuing to beat.
2 teaspoons baking powder	
1 teaspoon baking soda	*5* Beat the cream cheese into the mixture.
3 tablespoons skim milk	
2 teaspoons powdered instant coffee	*6* Sift the flour, baking powder, and baking soda into the mixture.
3½ tablespoons toasted chia seeds (see the following Tip)	*7* In a small saucepan over medium heat, heat the milk to lukewarm, and dissolve the coffee in the milk.
	8 Mix the coffee into the wet mixture.
	9 Add the chia seeds to the mixture, and mix until well combined.
	10 Pour the mixture into the muffin tin.
	11 Bake for 15 minutes.

Per serving: Calories 165 (From Fat 57); Fat 7g (Saturated 1g); Cholesterol 16mg; Sodium 173mg; Carbohydrate 23g (Dietary Fiber 1g); Protein 3g.

Note: When adding dairy products, do so slowly to prevent them from coming apart.

Tip: To toast chia seeds, place the seeds in a frying pan over low heat. Stir the chia constantly for up to 10 minutes, until the seeds are toasted evenly; remove from the heat.

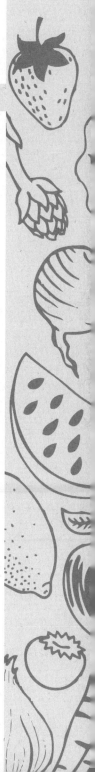

Chia Chocolate and Walnut Muffins

Prep time: 30 min • **Cook time:** 15 min • **Yield:** 12 servings

Ingredients	Directions
1 egg	*1* Preheat the oven to 350 degrees and line a muffin tin with 12 liners.
2 egg whites	
6 tablespoons sugar	*2* In a large bowl, beat the egg, egg whites, and sugar until almost white.
3½ tablespoons sunflower oil	
⅓ cup fat-free vanilla yogurt	*3* Slowly add the oil.
7 tablespoons skim milk	
2 teaspoons vanilla extract	*4* Add the yogurt, milk, and vanilla extract.
1¾ cups flour	
2 teaspoons baking powder	*5* In a separate bowl, sift the flour and baking powder.
1 ounce unsweetened cocoa powder	*6* Add the dry ingredients to the wet ingredients and mix until well combined.
½ cup walnuts, broken	
5 tablespoons milled chia seeds	*7* Add the cocoa powder, walnuts, and chia and mix until well combined.
	8 Pour the mixture into the muffin tin.
	9 Bake for 15 minutes.

Per serving: Calories 191 (From Fat 75); Fat 8g (Saturated 1g); Cholesterol 16mg; Sodium 92mg; Carbohydrate 25g (Dietary Fiber 3g); Protein 5g.

Vary It! In this recipe we use walnuts, but you can use any nuts that you like.

Banana Chia Muffins

Prep time: 15 min • **Cook time:** 15 min • **Yield:** 12 servings

Ingredients	Directions
2 bananas	*1* Preheat the oven to 400 degrees and line a muffin tin with 12 liners.
4 tablespoons milled chia seeds	
6 tablespoons unrefined sugar	*2* Cut the bananas in very small pieces and coat the pieces in the chia. Set aside.
1 egg	
1 egg white	*3* In a mixer, beat the sugar, egg, and egg white.
4 tablespoons sunflower oil	*4* Slowly add the oil.
7 tablespoons skim milk	
¼ cup lowfat cream cheese	*5* Add the milk, cream cheese, and vanilla extract.
1 teaspoon vanilla extract	
1¾ cups flour	*6* In a medium bowl, sift the flour and baking powder; add the oats and nuts and combine.
3 teaspoons baking powder	
⅔ cup medium rolled oats	*7* Add the dry ingredients to the wet ingredients.
½ cup whole nuts of your choice	*8* Pour half of the muffin mixture into the muffin tin. Cover the mixture with half of the chia-coated bananas. Cover the bananas with the remaining muffin mixture. Top with the remaining bananas, slightly pushing the bananas into the muffin mixture.
	9 Bake for 15 minutes.

Per serving: Calories 223 (From Fat 86); Fat 10g (Saturated 2g); Cholesterol 18mg; Sodium 139mg; Carbohydrate 30g (Dietary Fiber 3g); Protein 5g.

Vary It! You can use pears or another other similar-textured fruit instead of bananas.

Celebratory Cakes

People celebrate special occasions with different types of cakes all over the world. Often, the recipes are handed down from grandparents to parents to children, and shared among family and friends. These traditional recipes can easily be enhanced nutritionally with chia seeds.

If one of your grandmother's recipes calls for any type of flour, simply reduce the amount of flour by the amount of milled chia seeds that you plan on adding. (We recommend adding ¼ cup of milled chia seeds to a typical cake recipe.) Then add the chia along with twice that amount of water (for example, if you add ¼ cup of milled chia, add ½ cup of water) to ensure that the consistency of the cake doesn't differ too much from what your grandma intended. This way, you can still enjoy her cake, but you're giving your family the extra nutrients from the chia seeds.

If you don't want to change the recipe for the batter of the cake, try adding chia as a topping. You can easily add whole chia seeds to any icing or fresh cream.

Whether it's a wedding in Spain, a graduation ceremony in the United States, Christmas in England, or a birthday party in Australia, chances are, cake will be served at some stage. More often then not, people love to indulge in cakes at any family celebration. So, why not treat your guests to a chia-spiked cake full of nutrients that still tastes fantastic? When you let out the secret that the cake you're serving is high in omega-3 fatty acids, fiber, protein, and antioxidants, you can bet people will want the recipe!

Chia Angel Food Cake with Lavender Icing

Prep time: 25 min • **Cook time:** 50 min • **Yield:** 12 servings

Ingredients	Directions
12 egg whites	**1** Preheat the oven to 325 degrees. Line a 9½-inch tube pan with parchment paper.
Pinch of cream of tartar	
1¼ cups granulated sugar	**2** In a medium bowl, beat the egg whites and cream of tartar until foamy. Sprinkle the sugar into the bowl, and continue beating until a soft meringue forms. Do not overbeat.
¾ cup cake flour	
3 tablespoons cornstarch	
5 tablespoons milled chia seeds	**3** In a mixer, place the flour, cornstarch, and chia seeds. Process until a smooth powder is obtained.
Lavender Icing (see following recipe)	**4** Fold the dry ingredients into the egg whites in a few batches. Do not add all the dry ingredients at once. Spoon the mixture into the pan. Bake for 50 minutes, or until the upper part browns and a knife sliced into the cake comes out clean. Remove from the oven and place the pan upside down on a cake rack to cool. When the cake is at room temperature, remove the pan.
	5 Use a spoon to drizzle the Lavender Icing on the cake in a zigzag pattern.

Lavender Icing

1 or 2 drops lavender essence	**1** In a small bowl, mix the lavender essence and 1 tablespoon of the water.
1 to 1½ tablespoons boiling water	
1 cup super-fine sugar	**2** In a separate bowl, sift the sugar.
	3 Add the lavender mixture to the sugar, and stir until well combined and runny enough to drizzle. If it's too stiff, add a few more drops of the water.

Per serving: Calories 242 (From Fat 8); Fat 1g (Saturated 0g); Cholesterol 0mg; Sodium 56mg; Carbohydrate 55g (Dietary Fiber 1g); Protein 5g.

Chia and Banana Cake

Prep time: 30 min • **Cook time:** 40 min • **Yield:** 12 servings

Ingredients	Directions
6 tablespoons brown sugar	*1* Preheat the oven to 350 degrees. Spray parchment paper with vegetable oil spray, and line an 8-inch cake pan with the parchment paper.
7 teaspoons water	
1½ cups sliced banana	
2 tablespoons whole chia seeds	*2* In a small bowl, mix the brown sugar and the water to form a light brown caramel. Place the caramel on the bottom of the pan.
1 egg	
⅔ cup sugar	*3* Add the sliced bananas to the bottom of the pan, arranging them in a round shape. Then sprinkle the whole chia seeds over the bananas.
2½ tablespoons honey	
2½ tablespoons sunflower oil	
5 egg whites	*4* In a medium bowl, beat the whole egg with ⅓ cup of the sugar and all the honey, until patterns are formed in the mixture. Slowly add the oil.
Pinch of cream of tartar	
1⅓ cups flour	*5* In a separate bowl, beat the egg whites with the remaining ⅓ cup of sugar and the cream of tartar until peaks form.
2 teaspoons baking powder	
½ cup almond flour	*6* In a third bowl, sift the flour, baking powder, and almond flour.
5 tablespoons milled chia seeds	
	7 Combine the 2 egg mixtures in one bowl and add the dry ingredients. Mix until well combined.
	8 Pour one-third of the mixture on top of the bananas in the pan, sprinkle 2½ tablespoons of the milled chia seeds over the mixture, pour another third of the mixture into the pan, sprinkle with the remaining 2½ tablespoons of chia, and then pour the remaining mixture into the pan.
	9 Bake for 40 minutes, until the cake is golden.
	10 Remove the cake from pan while it's still warm, and let it sit to cool.

Per serving: Calories 225 (From Fat 63); Fat 7g (Saturated 1g); Cholesterol 15mg; Sodium 100mg; Carbohydrate 37g (Dietary Fiber 3g); Protein 5g.

Chia Chocolate Sponge Cake

Prep time: 25 min • **Cook time:** 45 min • **Yield:** 12 servings

Ingredients	*Directions*
1 egg	*1* Preheat the oven to 325 degrees. Line an angel food cake pan with parchment paper.
⅓ **cup water**	
1 cup sugar	*2* In a medium bowl, beat the whole egg and water with ½ cup of the sugar; add the oil very slowly and then add the vanilla extract.
⅓ **cup sunflower oil**	
1 teaspoon vanilla extract	
1⅓ cups cake flour	*3* In a separate bowl, sift the flour, baking powder, cocoa, and salt; add the milled chia seeds.
2 teaspoons baking powder	
6 tablespoons unsweetened cocoa powder	*4* In a third bowl, whip the egg whites with the remaining ½ cup of sugar until a meringue forms.
½ **teaspoon salt**	
7 tablespoons milled chia seeds	*5* Mix all three bowls together by adding the second and third bowls into the first. Mix everything together until well combined.
6 egg whites	
	6 Pour the mixture into the pan.
	7 Bake for 45 minutes, until a knife sliced into the cake comes out clean.
	8 Remove from the oven, and place the pan upside down on a cake rack to cool. When the cake is at room temperature, remove the pan.

Per serving: Calories 212 (From Fat 71); Fat 8g (Saturated 1g); Cholesterol 16mg; Sodium 199mg; Carbohydrate 32g (Dietary Fiber 2g); Protein 5g.

Chia Orange Sponge Cake

Prep time: 15 min • **Cook time:** 35 min • **Yield:** 12 servings

Ingredients	Directions
1 egg	**1** Preheat the oven to 325 degrees. Line an angel food cake pan with parchment paper.
5 egg whites	
¾ cup sugar	**2** In a medium bowl, beat the egg, 2 of the egg whites, and 6 tablespoons of the sugar until patterns made with the whisk keep a firm shape.
⅓ cup sunflower oil	
2 tablespoons grated orange rind	**3** Very slowly add the oil.
⅓ cup fresh orange juice	**4** Add the orange rind and orange juice.
1⅔ cups cake flour	**5** In a separate bowl, sift the flour and the baking powder.
2 teaspoons baking powder	
Pinch of cream of tartar	**6** In a third bowl, whisk the remaining 3 egg whites with the cream of tartar; add the remaining 6 tablespoons of sugar, and continue beating until peaks form.
4 tablespoons whole chia seeds	
	7 Combine the egg whites mixture with the beaten eggs mixture and mix slowly.
	8 Fold the dry ingredients into the wet while adding the chia seeds little by little.
	9 Pour the mixture into the pan.
	10 Bake for 35 minutes, until a knife sliced into the cake comes out clean.
	11 Remove from the oven, and place the pan upside down on a cake rack to cool. When the cake is at room temperature, remove the pan.

Per serving: Calories 205 (From Fat 68); Fat 8g (Saturated 1g); Cholesterol 16mg; Sodium 97mg; Carbohydrate 30g (Dietary Fiber 2g); Protein 4g.

Vary It! Take out the orange peel and orange juice, and you have a good basic sponge cake recipe. From there, you can add different flavors, like lemon, pineapple, and so on.

Chia and Walnut Sponge Cake

Prep time: 25 min • **Cook time:** 40 min • **Yield:** 12 servings

Ingredients	Directions
1 egg	**1** Preheat the oven to 325 degrees.
6 egg whites	**2** In a medium bowl, beat the egg, 2 of the egg whites, ⅓ cup of the sugar, and the honey until creamy. Slowly add the oil.
⅔ cup sugar	
2½ tablespoons honey	
3½ tablespoons sunflower oil	**3** In a separate bowl, whip the remaining 4 egg whites with the remaining ⅓ cup of sugar and the cream of tartar until peaks form.
Pinch of cream of tartar	
1⅔ cups cake flour	**4** In a third bowl, sift the flour and baking powder.
2 teaspoons baking powder	
5 tablespoons milled chia seeds	**5** In a blender, finely chop the walnuts. Add 1 tablespoon of the flour while blending.
⅓ cup whole walnuts	**6** Slowly add the beaten egg mixture into the egg white mixture and then slowly fold in the dry ingredients.
1 tablespoon powdered sugar, for garnish	
	7 Add the chia and walnuts to the mixture.
	8 Pour into an angel food cake pan and bake for approximately 40 minutes, until a knife sliced into the cake comes out clean.
	9 Remove from the oven, and place the pan upside down on a cake rake to cool. When the cake is at room temperature, remove the pan.
	10 Dust the cake with powdered sugar.

Per serving: Calories 208 (From Fat 63); Fat 7g (Saturated 1g); Cholesterol 16mg; Sodium 101mg; Carbohydrate 32g (Dietary Fiber 1g); Protein 5g.

More Sweets Treats

It's not just after dinner or at parties that we crave sweet things. For some people, their treat of choice may be a cookie or a chocolate bar. Whatever your indulgent treat is, there's always a way to make it a bit more nutritious using chia seeds. And that's what this section is all about — some more sweet treats tricked out with chia to be enjoyed at any time.

Why home-baked goodies beat the rest

If you're going to treat yourself to a sugary snack — whether at a party or at home — at least make your own. The ones available in stores are processed and full of additives and ingredients that you can't even pronounce.

Here's why you should be baking your own treats:

✔ **You can choose your own ingredients.** Having control over all the ingredients means you can pick good-quality flours, the freshest produce, and organic foods if that's important to you. You can also choose healthier versions of foods — such as stevia instead of sugar, lowfat milk instead of whole milk, or gluten-free ingredients if you desire.

✔ **You can control portion sizes.** If you bake a cake or a sheet of brownies, you can cut it into individual portions that are small enough to satisfy your sweet craving but not so big that you eat more than half the calories you need in a day. (Have you seen the size of some of those bakery treats?)

✔ **You can save money.** Baking your own treats is much cheaper than buying from the store. Just make sure your pantry is well stocked with the basic ingredients needed for baking.

Chia Meringues

Prep time: 30 min • **Cook time:** 1½–3 hr • **Yield:** 20 servings

Ingredients	Directions
3 egg whites	*1* Preheat the oven to 200 degrees. Line a 12-x-16-inch baking pan with parchment paper.
Pinch of cream of tartar	
¼ cup walnuts	*2* In a medium bowl, beat the egg whites with the cream of tartar until it's foamy; set aside.
13 tablespoons powdered sugar	
2 tablespoons cornstarch	*3* In a food processor, blend the walnuts.
4 tablespoons milled chia seeds	*4* In another bowl, mix the walnuts with the powdered sugar, cornstarch, chia, and super-fine sugar.
½ cup super-fine sugar	*5* Add the egg mixture to the walnut mixture, folding it in very gently.
	6 Place the mixture in an icing bag with a rippled nozzle. Pipe the mixture on the pan with peaks.
	7 Bake from 90 to 180 minutes, until the meringues have formed.
	8 Turn off the oven and allow the meringues to cool in the oven, about 30 minutes. Remove from the oven and slide them off the parchment paper, taking care not to break them.
	9 Store in airtight container for up to 14 days.

Per serving: Calories 57 (From Fat 11); Fat 1g (Saturated 0g); Cholesterol 0mg; Sodium 9mg; Carbohydrate 11g (Dietary Fiber 1g); Protein 1g.

Vary It! To make a cake out of this meringue, whip some full-fat cream until it forms stiff peaks. Then spread it evenly over the meringue base. Add some fresh fruits such as peach slices or strawberries and raspberries, and sprinkle with grated chocolate. This is a deliciously fresh and light dessert that most people will love!

Chia Brownies

Prep time: 20 min • **Cook time:** 40 min • **Yield:** 16 servings

Ingredients	Directions
7 tablespoons margarine	**1** Preheat the oven to 350 degrees.
6 tablespoons powdered sugar	**2** In a large bowl, beat the margarine and powdered sugar until creamy. Add the whole egg and egg whites one by one.
1 egg	
2 egg whites	
1 cup flour	**3** In a separate large bowl, sift the flour and cocoa; add the milled chia and combine.
4 tablespoons unsweetened cocoa powder	
6 tablespoons milled chia seeds	**4** Add the dry ingredients to the wet ingredients and mix well. This is the brownie mixture.
7 ounces lowfat cream cheese	**5** In a third large bowl, beat the cream cheese and sugar until creamy. Add the chia jam. This is the filling.
¼ cup sugar	
5 tablespoons chia jam (see Chapter 13 for recipes)	**6** Spray a tempered glass pan with vegetable oil spray.
	7 Pour half the brownie mixture into the pan.
	8 Spread the filling over it; cover with the remaining brownie mixture.
	9 Bake for 25 minutes.
	10 Remove from the oven and let cool. Then cut into squares.

Per serving: Calories 151 (From Fat 81); Fat 9g (Saturated 3g); Cholesterol 21mg; Sodium 99mg; Carbohydrate 15g (Dietary Fiber 2g); Protein 4g.

Chia Cookies

Prep time: 20 min • **Cook time:** 15–20 min • **Yield:** 15 servings

Ingredients	Directions
¾ cup flour	**1** Preheat the oven to 400 degrees.
3 teaspoons baking powder	**2** In a medium bowl, sift the flour and baking powder.
¾ cup unrefined sugar	**3** Add the sugar and margarine to the bowl and mix well using a hand mixer, or mix in a food processor.
⅔ cup butter	
1 egg	**4** In a separate bowl, beat the egg, egg white, and honey.
1 egg white	
1 tablespoon honey	**5** Add this egg mixture to the sugar, margarine, and flour, and mix well to form a soft dough.
5 tablespoons milled chia seeds	
2 tablespoons sugar	**6** Gather the dough, wrap it in plastic, and leave it in the refrigerator for at least 30 minutes.
	7 Roll out the dough until it's thin. Sprinkle the dough with chia, fold it in 3, and cool again.
	8 Roll out the dough to around ¼ inch thick; cut the desired cookie shapes.
	9 Place the cookie shapes on a baking pan and sprinkle with the sugar.
	10 Bake for 15 to 20 minutes, or until golden brown.

Per serving: Calories 160 (From Fat 82); Fat 9g (Saturated 5g); Cholesterol 34mg; Sodium 90mg; Carbohydrate 18g (Dietary Fiber 1g); Protein 2g.

Vary It! This dough can be rolled into a roll and then cut into sticks. Make a hole in the middle and fill with chia jam (see Chapter 13 for recipes). Close the hole, and bake as above.

Part V
The Part of Tens

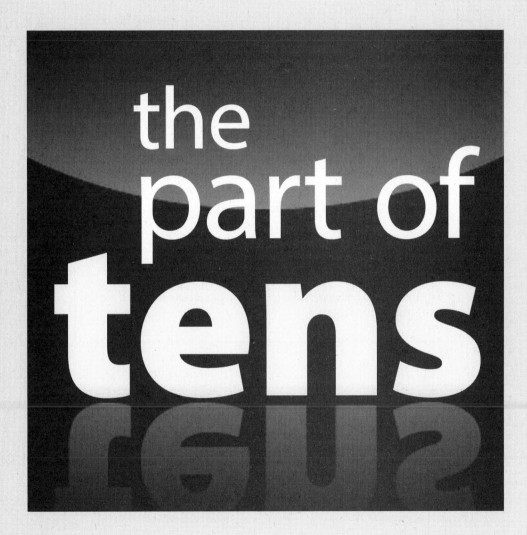

For ten facts you probably didn't know about chia, head to www.dummies.com/extras/cookingwithchia.

In this part . . .

- ✔ Incorporate chia into your daily routine by making quick changes to your diet.
- ✔ See why chia is such an amazing superfood.
- ✔ Use chia to boost the nutrients in your kids' meals without their suspecting a thing.

Chapter 16

Ten Tricks for Getting Chia into Your Everyday Diet

*T*ossing some chia seeds into whatever you're eating is a wonderful way to boost the nutritional value of your meals. The seeds are tiny and have virtually no flavor, but they're brimming with nutrients! So, you can simply add chia seeds to your meals to gain numerous health benefits, without altering the flavor of your favorite foods. They require no preparation, are eaten raw, and are the perfect accompaniment to any meal.

A great way to help your family improve their diets is to keep a bag of chia seeds on the kitchen table so they're always reminded to just add chia!

In this chapter, we give you ten easy ways to add chia to your diet.

Add It to Your Morning Cereal

Whether you like bran flakes, oatmeal, or granola, simply add 2 tablespoons of whole chia seeds to your favorite breakfast cereal, and you'll benefit from the added energy you'll get throughout the day. For more chia breakfast ideas, check out Chapter 6.

Stir It into Yogurt

Yogurt is a tasty snack any time of day. Whether you enjoy probiotic yogurt (with live cultures) or you go for more of a sugar-loaded, less-healthy yogurt option, by adding whole chia seeds to this delicious snack, you can be sure you're hitting your omega-3, fiber, and protein requirements for the day. We think yogurt is a great way to get chia into your day, and we've put together some delicious recipes using yogurt in Chapter 6.

Sneak It into Your Sandwiches

Who doesn't love the convenience of a sandwich for lunch? With so many combinations, you can enjoy a mix of salads, meats, spreads, or just plain jelly. Whatever you choose to put between your favorite slices of bread or in a wrap, simply sprinkle some whole chia seeds over your creation to add valuable nutrients to your lunchtime favorite.

Eat It Straight Up

If you enjoy the crunch of chia, simply eat the seeds as they are! Store the seeds in a small canister, and you can bring them anywhere. Then, when you feel the need, munch away to get extra energy and nutrition. Eating whole chia seeds is a great way to stay energized on long runs or hikes, or while doing any type of exercise where you need to keep your energy levels up.

If you eat the seeds as they are, make sure to drink a glass of water either before or after. Chia seeds absorb liquid and if no water is available, they'll absorb your stomach juices, which can lead to a stomachache.

Toss It Over Salads

Sometimes a simple salad is all you have time for at lunch or dinner, so load your salads with extra nutrients, sprinkle some whole chia seeds over them. Try ditching the chicken or beef you usually add to your salads, and get your protein fix from chia, which has all the essential amino acids, making it a complete protein — a rare find in the plant world!

Mix It into Your Favorite Dips

Dips are a delicious snack to enjoy anytime, whether you serve them with chips, carrot sticks, or celery. When you add chia seeds to your dips, you can lessen the guilt by knowing that you're adding healthy fats, a complete protein, and much needed fiber. Some of our favorites to add chia to are guacamole, hummus, salsa, sour cream, and nut butters.

To add chia to any of your favorite dips, simply make some chia gel by mixing six parts water with one part whole chia seeds, and let them sit for ten minutes, stirring occasionally. Then add the chia gel to your favorite dip.

Stir It into Water or Juice

If you're in a real rush, simply add some whole chia seeds to a glass of water or juice, stir well, and drink fast before it thickens up and becomes a chia gel. If you're the type of person who thrives on healthy habits, drinking back a shot of chia water every morning is a fantastic routine to get into without adding any extra calories to your day!

Mix It into Salad Dressing

Dressing a salad can turn boring greens into mouthwatering meals. To make a simple but delicious salad dressing, try mixing 6 tablespoons olive oil, 2 tablespoon balsamic vinegar, ½ teaspoon mustard, ½ teaspoon honey, and 1 teaspoon milled chia seeds. Mix well and pour over salad leaves to turn your everyday salads into delicious meals full of essential nutrients.

Add It to Soups

A hot bowl of soup made with fresh vegetables is the ultimate healthy lunch, and chia seeds are the perfect addition. Not only do they thicken any soup recipe, but they add quality protein and healthy fats to the already nutritious bowl of blended or chunky vegetables.

To add chia seeds to soups, mix whole chia seeds with six parts water and leave it to sit for ten minutes to form a gel. Then stir this gel into the soup. Or easier still, use milled chia seeds, and you can stir them right into the soup and thicken it up. Check out Chapter 9 for some tasty soup recipes you're sure to enjoy.

Sprinkle It on Peanut Butter and Banana Toast

A delicious and quick way to get the benefit of chia into your diet is to spread some peanut butter over a slice of whole-grain toast, add sliced banana, and drizzle with honey. Then sprinkle some whole chia seeds over everything. This simple recipe is a great breakfast to set you up for the day or as an any-time snack to enjoy when you need energy!

Chapter 17

Ten Ways Chia Is a Superfood

In This Chapter

▶ Identifying the essential nutrients found in chia

▶ Homing in on the heart-healthy benefits of chia

▶ Discovering chia's unique properties

Chia is one of the most nutrient-dense foods found anywhere in the world. Not only is it exceptionally high in essential nutrients such as protein and fiber, but chia benefits your health by giving you the vitamins, minerals, and antioxidants necessary for good health.

Chia seeds have a lot to boast about, including their ease of use, long shelf life, and many more properties that make it a true superfood. You'll find it hard to track down a more complete food that is so easy to add to all your favorite meals, increasing your diet's nutritional value and helping to improve your health and well-being.

Chia Is an Excellent Plant Source of Omega-3 Fatty Acids

People everywhere are becoming more aware of the fact that we need omega-3 fatty acids for our brains to function well, our hearts to pump strong, and more. Now, thanks to chia, you can easily get enough of this all-important nutrient. When it comes to plants, chia is one of the best sources of omega-3s. Plus, because chia is a *renewable resource* — a plant that can be grown and harvested and replanted again — you can be confident that you aren't diminishing the world fish supplies to get your omega-3 fix.

Chia Is a Complete Protein

Chia seeds are a source of high-quality protein that our bodies need to build and replace body cells. The protein in chia contains all nine essential amino acids, which makes it a complete protein. This is why chia is especially fantastic for vegans and vegetarians — finding a source of complete protein in the plant kingdom is difficult, but chia provides just that, a complete protein suitable for vegan and vegetarian diets.

Chia Has Both Soluble and Insoluble Fiber

Chia is high in fiber, but what gives chia the edge is that it has both soluble *and* insoluble fiber. Soluble fiber mixes with water, swelling to make you feel fuller longer. It also slows digestion and helps to balance blood sugar levels and lower cholesterol levels. Insoluble fiber doesn't mix with water; it provides bulk in the diet, helping to keep you regular and prevent constipation. Both types of fiber are essential for a balanced diet.

Chia Is Gluten-Free

Many gluten-free foods contain unhealthy additives, undermining your efforts to choose healthy, gluten-free products. With chia, you get a naturally gluten-free food without the nasty additives. This means you can choose chia that's packed full of essential nutrients while cutting down on processed gluten-free foods.

You may have heard more and more people talking lately about "going gluten-free." Gluten is a protein derived from wheat. Some people — those with celiac disease or wheat allergy — need to avoid gluten. But many people without these special conditions also benefit from reducing or eliminating gluten from their diets. To learn more about gluten-free diets, check out *Living Gluten-Free For Dummies,* 2nd Edition, by Danna Korn (Wiley), or the variety of gluten-free cookbooks in the *For Dummies* series. Just go to Dummies.com and search for "gluten."

Chia Absorbs Liquids

Chia seeds are *hydrophilic,* meaning that when mixed with water or any other liquids, the seeds absorb the liquid and swell to up to ten times their size. This helps you feel fuller longer, helping you eat less and maintain a healthy weight. It also forms a physical barrier, slowing your body's absorption of carbohydrates, which help to balance blood sugar levels. This gives people who have diabetes a natural way to help manage their blood sugar.

Your Body Can Easily Absorb Chia's Nutrients

The shells of chia seeds are very soft, so when you eat a whole chia seed, your body quickly breaks down the shell and easily absorbs all the nutrients contained within the shell. This is very different from other seeds high in omega-3s, such as flaxseeds. Flaxseeds have very hard shells; when you eat them whole, your body can't break down the shells, so the whole seed, with the precious omega-3s and other nutrients contained within it, just pass through the body undigested. In order for your body to get the benefits from the nutrients in flax, the seeds must be broken down manually before being eaten — so you need to grind all flaxseeds or buy seeds that are already ground so your body can absorb the nutrients. That's why chia is so great! You don't need to grind them — your body can easily absorb the essential nutrients within chia's soft shell.

Chia Helps Protect Your Heart

Not only does chia help reduce blood pressure, but it has been shown to reduce cholesterol because of its high concentrations of omega-3s. Chia has enough alpha-linolenic acid (ALA; see Chapter 2) to help maintain normal blood cholesterol levels, in addition to helping reduce the risk of cardiovascular disease.

Chia Is Easy to Use

The subtle taste of chia seeds means that you can add it to all your favorite foods without affecting the taste, which makes it easy to use in everyday meals and snacks. You don't need to cook chia seeds — in fact, they're best eaten raw — so there is no preparation time. Simply toss some seeds into your foods to benefit from all chia has to offer.

Chia seeds have a shelf life of up to five years from harvest and can be kept at room temperature — no special storage requirements. This makes them convenient to keep for long periods of time. You can simply open a bag of chia, leave it on the kitchen table, and add it to everything — couldn't be easier!

Chia Is Loaded with Antioxidants

One of the unique properties that make chia seeds a superfood is the fact that chia is so high in natural antioxidants. These antioxidants help to reduce oxidative stress and help to prevent the onset of common degenerative diseases. People need to increase the amount of antioxidants in their diets, and chia can do just that with its high level of antioxidants found naturally.

It's High in Magnesium, Selenium, and Zinc

Chia is high in zinc, which helps the immune system and nervous system function well. Magnesium is needed for almost all body functions, and it's also found in high quantities in chia seeds. Selenium, known for its role in thyroid and immune function, is found — you guessed it! — in chia. All three of these nutrients are necessary for good health, and chia is a fantastic way to get them into your diet.

Chapter 18

Ten Ways to Sneak Chia into Your Kids' Food

Kids can be tough customers to please, and when you're trying to get them to eat healthy, any tricks that boost the healthy foods in their diets are welcome! That's where chia seeds can lend a helping hand. Because cha is high in omega-3 fatty acids, fiber, protein, and many vitamins and minerals, if you can get your children to include chia in their daily diets, you're on the right road to healthy eating. The beauty of chia seeds is their subtle taste, so you can easily add them to kids' meals and they won't know the difference.

The tips in this chapter give you an idea of how to get your fussy eaters eating chia seeds despite themselves, so you can be happy in the knowledge that some valuable nutrients are making it into those little bodies.

Blend Chia into Smoothies

Kids love smoothies! They taste great and are fun to make. If your child turns up her nose at vegetables, you can put them in a smoothie mixed with some sweet fruits, and she'll likely lap up your concoction. To make the smoothie even better, just add milled chia seeds to the blender — most children won't even know they're eating well. To learn all about smoothies and get some smoothie recipes, check out Chapter 8.

Milled chia is just whole chia seeds that have been ground down into a powdery texture so they retain all their nutrients. You can buy chia that has already been milled — it's sometimes called *ground chia* — or you can grind chia yourself in a coffee grinder.

Sprinkle Chia into Cereal

Many kids start their days with their favorite breakfast cereals. Usually, getting them to eat cereals isn't a struggle, so take this opportunity to spike your kids' cereal with a spoonful of chia seeds. You can usually get away with using the tiny whole seeds, because they blend in well with most cereals, but if your little ones start to object, use milled chia instead — you can mix it in, so it completely disappears within the cereal.

Hide Chia in Pasta Sauce

Pasta is a family favorite. To make it more nutritious, mix milled chia seeds into your favorite pasta sauce just before mixing it into the pasta. The kids will never notice the difference.

You can make a delicious but simple pasta sauce by frying a chopped onion in a little olive oil and then adding a can of chopped tomatoes, some finely sliced bell peppers, a handful of sliced mushrooms, and some dried marjoram. Simmer the ingredients together for 15 minutes or so, and then blend the mixture before adding milled chia seeds and serving with pasta. For more great recipes that kids love, check out Chapter 12.

Sprinkle Chia over Pizza

We can't think of a kid who doesn't love pizza. You can capitalize on your kids' pizza obsession by sneaking some chia into the mix.

For a quick pizza, spread small round pita breads with some tomato paste. Top with grated cheese, fresh tomatoes, sliced onion, and pepperoni slices. Put them under the broiler for five minutes and, just before serving, sprinkle some whole chia seeds over each pizza. This is a perfect way to satisfy hungry kids while making sure they get enough nutrients!

Mix Chia into Baby-Food Purees

When you begin to wean your baby from an all-milk diet, it's hard to figure out what foods to feed her that will meet her nutritional requirements. Chia seeds are an excellent source of omega-3s (see Chapter 2), and babies need omega-3s for brain development. Simply add milled chia to your baby's fruit and vegetable purees to help her get what she needs to outsmart you someday.

Stir Chia through Scrambled Eggs

Scrambled eggs are a favorite for toddlers and kids of all ages, and they're easy to prepare, too, so parents are often big fans! Although eggs provide lots of great nutrients, to make them even *more* nutritious, simply add milled chia seeds to the beaten eggs before cooking, and mix well. For some more tasty egg recipes that your kids may like to try, turn to Chapter 7.

Add Them to Yummy Yogurts

Most kids love yogurt, so next time your little one is crying out for a yummy yogurt treat, mix in some chia seeds before handing that container over. If he doesn't mind the added texture, you can use whole chia seeds. If he screams, "What's that?!" simply use milled chia seeds, and he won't be able to detect any difference. For more yummy yogurt recipes for your kids to try, check out Chapter 6.

 Instead of sneaking the chia into the yogurt (or any food, really), you can try making it a game: Just start calling chia seeds "sprinkles," and let your kids sprinkle them on top of yogurt, fruit, or anything else. Sprinkles sound a whole lot more fun (and tastier) to kids than chia seeds do, and who cares what you call them? The nutrients are the same!

Make Chia Fruit Ice Popsicles

Popsicles are a big favorite with kids, and the good news is: They're easy to make and can be very healthy. All you have to do is blend up some fruits (for example, bananas, strawberries, raspberries, and blueberries) and add some water. Then mix in some milled chia seeds. It's sort of like a smoothie, but the fun part is to pour this smoothie mixture into popsicle trays and stick them in the freezer. When your kids are asking for a treat, you can pull out one these delicious-tasting, refreshing popsicles and know they're getting a nutritious snack.

Add Chia to Apple Crumble

To add extra nutrients to your favorite apple crumble dessert recipe, simply add whole chia seeds to the crumble part of the recipe before baking. You can add chia to any crumble recipe, so if blackberries are in season or your kids are fans of rhubarb, go ahead and add chia to the mix. You won't feel so guilty about giving your kids dessert if you know it's loaded with nutrients from chia!

Sneak Chia into Rice Krispies Treats

Rice Krispies Treats are as much a part of childhood as skinned knees and whining, "Are we there yet?" Why not boost the nutritional value of these chewy treats with chia? Just add it to the mix along with the cereal. For more chia-infused kid treats, check out Chapter 12.

Metric Conversion Guide

· ·

Note: The recipes in this book weren't developed or tested using metric measurements. There may be some variation in quality when converting to metric units.

Common Abbreviations

Abbreviation(s)	What It Stands For
cm	Centimeter
C., c.	Cup
G, g	Gram
kg	Kilogram
L, l	Liter
lb.	Pound
mL, ml	Milliliter
oz.	Ounce
pt.	Pint
t., tsp.	Teaspoon
T., Tb., Tbsp.	Tablespoon

Volume

U.S. Units	Canadian Metric	Australian Metric
¼ teaspoon	1 milliliter	1 milliliter
½ teaspoon	2 milliliters	2 milliliters
1 teaspoon	5 milliliters	5 milliliters
1 tablespoon	15 milliliters	20 milliliters
¼ cup	50 milliliters	60 milliliters

(continued)

Volume *(continued)*

U.S. Units	*Canadian Metric*	*Australian Metric*
⅓ cup	75 milliliters	80 milliliters
½ cup	125 milliliters	125 milliliters
⅔ cup	150 milliliters	170 milliliters
¾ cup	175 milliliters	190 milliliters
1 cup	250 milliliters	250 milliliters
1 quart	1 liter	1 liter
1½ quarts	1.5 liters	1.5 liters
2 quarts	2 liters	2 liters
2½ quarts	2.5 liters	2.5 liters
3 quarts	3 liters	3 liters
4 quarts (1 gallon)	4 liters	4 liters

Weight

U.S. Units	*Canadian Metric*	*Australian Metric*
1 ounce	30 grams	30 grams
2 ounces	55 grams	60 grams
3 ounces	85 grams	90 grams
4 ounces (¼ pound)	115 grams	125 grams
8 ounces (½ pound)	225 grams	225 grams
16 ounces (1 pound)	455 grams	500 grams (½ kilogram)

Length

Inches	*Centimeters*
0.5	1.5
1	2.5
2	5.0
3	7.5
4	10.0
5	12.5
6	15.0

Inches	Centimeters
7	17.5
8	20.5
9	23.0
10	25.5
11	28.0
12	30.5

Temperature (Degrees)

Fahrenheit	Celsius
32	0
212	100
250	120
275	140
300	150
325	160
350	180
375	190
400	200
425	220
450	230
475	240
500	260

Index

About the Authors

Barrie Rogers: Barrie's journey with chia began in December 2008 when he hurt his back while on vacation in Florida. He was supposed to play golf with a guy he had never met before, but he had to cancel the game because of the pain in his back. His golf partner called Barrie and gave him some chia because he thought it might help. After taking the chia, Barrie felt relief from his back pain within two days and was so impressed with the improvement that he met with the man who gave it to him and got more chia to bring home to Ireland. He shared the chia seeds among his family and friends who were suffering from various health issues, and their feedback was very positive. Unfortunately, they couldn't continue using it because chia wasn't available in Ireland or Europe and there was very little knowledge about it at all. Barrie educated himself about chia and reached out to chia expert Dr. Wayne Coates to try find a way to bring chia to Ireland so that more people could benefit from the tiny seeds.

In late 2009, Barrie formed a company with Ray Owens called Chia bia (www. chiabia.com), and they continued on an amazing journey to bring them to where they are now: the leading suppliers of chia to the European market. The work they've done with Dr. Coates ensures that the chia seeds supplied by Chia bia are of the highest quality, and they're continuing their efforts to raise awareness about the benefits of chia so that more people can enhance their well-being with chia.

Before this journey, Barrie worked as a financial advisor for several years. Prior to that, he worked in the manufacturing industry for over ten years, seven of which were with Intel in a training and development capacity.

Debbie Dooly: Debbie's journey with chia began when she started working with Barrie and Ray at Chia bia and discovered the benefits of chia for herself. Having traveled extensively throughout China, Southeast Asia, Australia, New Zealand, and many parts of South America prior to working for Chia bia, Debbie developed a keen interest in local foods, healthy eating, and healthy cooking. Debbie is passionate about including chia in her diet and feels it has benefited both her and her young family. In addition to her general well-being improving while using chia, the big difference was obvious throughout her pregnancies. Before she found chia, during her first pregnancy, she lacked energy and felt tired. But when she carried her second son, after making chia a part of her life, she felt full of energy, which she attributes to the inclusion of chia in her diet. Debbie is now International Marketing Manager for Chia bia and is living the chia way of life. She's eager to share her experiences with as many people as possible, so that more people can discover the benefits of chia for themselves. Debbie lives in County Waterford in Ireland with her partner, Donny, and their two sons, Finn and Seán.

Dedication

I would like to dedicate this book to Lucky Luke O'Loughlin. If he had not taken the time to introduce chia to me, the journey I am on would not have happened.

—Barrie Rogers

Authors' Acknowledgments

We would like to thank Tracy Boggier, Elizabeth Kuball, and the entire team at John Wiley & Sons, who gave us the opportunity to write about chia and showed us great support and guidance throughout the process. Thanks also to Rachel Nix, our technical editor; Emily Nolan, who tested all our recipes; Patty Santelli, our nutrition analyst; and photographer T. J. Hine, all of whom contributed greatly to the making of this book. We would also like to thank Pat Moore, our talented photographer, who worked with us to make some fantastic photos for some of the recipes we've created.

Barrie Rogers: The journey over the past six years from my introduction to chia is in no small part thanks to the great work of Dr. Wayne Coates, who has dedicated over 20 years of his life to chia. His guidance, honesty, and passion for chia since I first reached out to him can never be underestimated. Not only have I gotten the opportunity to meet somebody who is focused on introducing more people to quality, affordable chia that can lead to better health and well-being, but I also have been very lucky to have formed a great friendship. I would also like to thank everybody who has supported me in any way and to say how lucky I am to have that support, especially from my wife, Sinéad, and kids, Vera and Finn, family, friends, and the team at Chia bia. I would like to thank Vilma La Presti, whose recipes have inspired some of my baking over the past several years. Last, I have to thank Debbie, my co-author — her efforts and her patience to understand my work have not gone unnoticed. It was a pleasure to work with you — and next time I bring an opportunity like this to you, I won't mind rejection. You're a saint!

Debbie Dooly: I'd really like to thank Barrie and Ray for introducing me to chia and employing me at Chia bia. What I've learned about chia has benefited my whole family. I would especially like to thank Dr. Wayne Coates for all the knowledge he has shared with us from his dedicated research into chia seeds. Barrie, thanks so much for giving me the opportunity to co-author this book — I've enjoyed it all, especially the chance to develop and share our delicious recipes and our knowledge of chia. Thanks also to all my family, especially my partner, Donny, and our children, Finn and Seán. And to everyone who has shown me support and tasted and given us feedback on our recipes, thank you.

Publisher's Acknowledgments

Senior Acquisitions Editor: Tracy Boggier

Project Editor: Elizabeth Kuball

Copy Editor: Elizabeth Kuball

Technical Editor: Kristina LaRue, RD, LD/N

Art Coordinator: Alicia B. South

Project Coordinator: Sheree Montgomery

Recipe Tester: Emily Nolan

Nutrition Analyst: Patricia Santelli

Photographers: T. J. Hines Photography, Pat Moore

Cover Image: Pat Moore

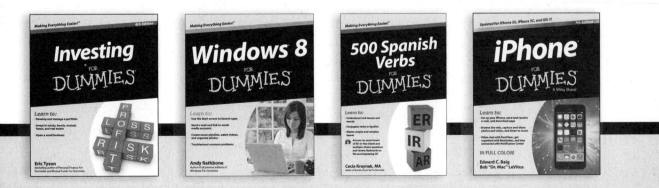

Math & Science

Algebra I For Dummies,
2nd Edition
978-0-470-55964-2

Anatomy and Physiology
For Dummies, 2nd Edition
978-0-470-92326-9

Astronomy For Dummies,
3rd Edition
978-1-118-37697-3

Biology For Dummies,
2nd Edition
978-0-470-59875-7

Chemistry For Dummies,
2nd Edition
978-1-118-00730-3

1001 Algebra II Practice
Problems For Dummies
978-1-118-44662-1

Microsoft Office

Excel 2013 For Dummies
978-1-118-51012-4

Office 2013 All-in-One
For Dummies
978-1-118-51636-2

PowerPoint 2013
For Dummies
978-1-118-50253-2

Word 2013 For Dummies
978-1-118-49123-2

Music

Blues Harmonica
For Dummies
978-1-118-25269-7

Guitar For Dummies,
3rd Edition
978-1-118-11554-1

iPod & iTunes
For Dummies, 10th Edition
978-1-118-50864-0

Programming

Beginning Programming
with C For Dummies
978-1-118-73763-7

Excel VBA Programming
For Dummies, 3rd Edition
978-1-118-49037-2

Java For Dummies,
6th Edition
978-1-118-40780-6

Religion & Inspiration

The Bible For Dummies
978-0-7645-5296-0

Buddhism For Dummies,
2nd Edition
978-1-118-02379-2

Catholicism For Dummies,
2nd Edition
978-1-118-07778-8

Self-Help & Relationships

Beating Sugar Addiction
For Dummies
978-1-118-54645-1

Meditation For Dummies,
3rd Edition
978-1-118-29144-3

Seniors

Laptops For Seniors
For Dummies, 3rd Edition
978-1-118-71105-7

Computers For Seniors
For Dummies, 3rd Edition
978-1-118-11553-4

iPad For Seniors
For Dummies, 6th Edition
978-1-118-72826-0

Social Security
For Dummies
978-1-118-20573-0

Smartphones & Tablets

Android Phones
For Dummies, 2nd Edition
978-1-118-72030-1

Nexus Tablets
For Dummies
978-1-118-77243-0

Samsung Galaxy S 4
For Dummies
978-1-118-64222-1

Samsung Galaxy Tabs
For Dummies
978-1-118-77294-2

Test Prep

ACT For Dummies,
5th Edition
978-1-118-01259-8

ASVAB For Dummies,
3rd Edition
978-0-470-63760-9

GRE For Dummies,
7th Edition
978-0-470-88921-3

Officer Candidate Tests
For Dummies
978-0-470-59876-4

Physician's Assistant Exam
For Dummies
978-1-118-11556-5

Series 7 Exam For Dummie
978-0-470-09932-2

Windows 8

Windows 8.1 All-in-One
For Dummies
978-1-118-82087-2

Windows 8.1 For Dummies
978-1-118-82121-3

Windows 8.1 For Dummies
Book + DVD Bundle
978-1-118-82107-7

Available in print and e-book formats.

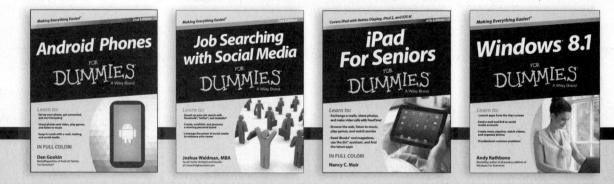

Available wherever books are sold. **For more information or to order direct visit www.dummies.com**

Take Dummies with you everywhere you go!

Whether you are excited about e-books, want more from the web, must have your mobile apps, or are swept up in social media, Dummies makes everything easier.

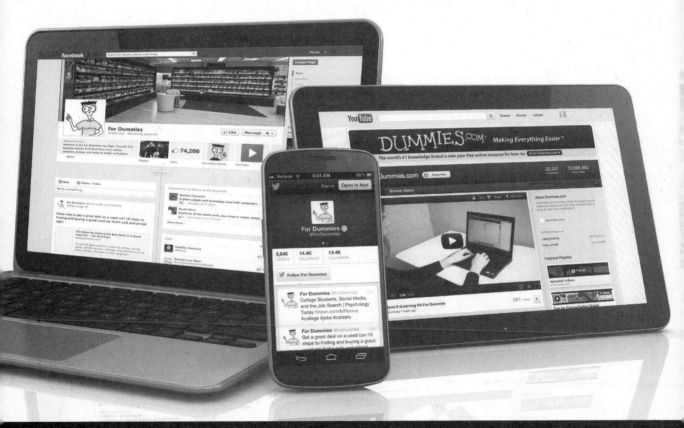

Leverage the Power

For Dummies is the global leader in the reference category and one of the most trusted and highly regarded brands in the world. No longer just focused on books, customers now have access to the For Dummies content they need in the format they want. Let us help you develop a solution that will fit your brand and help you connect with your customers.

Advertising & Sponsorships

Connect with an engaged audience on a powerful multimedia site, and position your message alongside expert how-to content.

Targeted ads • Video • Email marketing • Microsites • Sweepstakes sponsorship

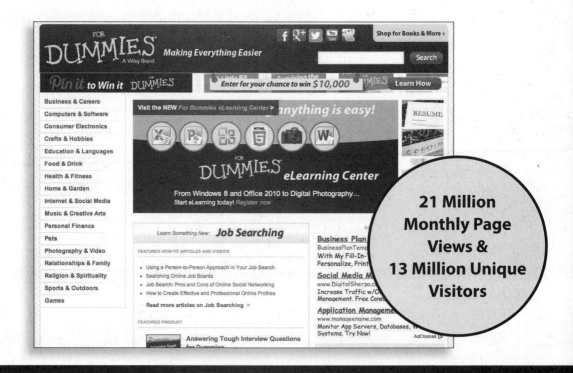

# of For Dummies

Custom Publishing

Reach a global audience in any language by creating a solution that will differentiate you from competitors, amplify your message, and encourage customers to make a buying decision.

Apps • Books • eBooks • Video • Audio • Webinars

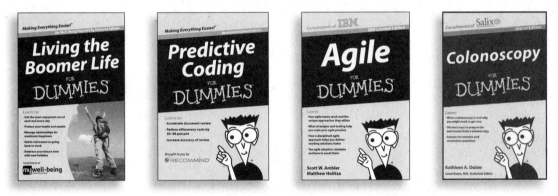

Brand Licensing & Content

Leverage the strength of the world's most popular reference brand to reach new audiences and channels of distribution.

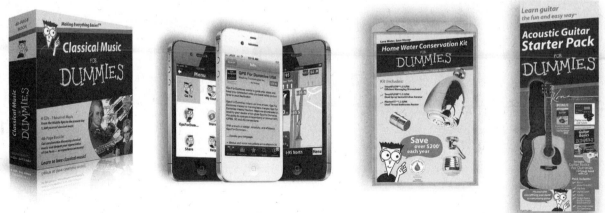

For more information, visit www.Dummies.com/biz

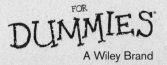

A Wiley Brand

Dummies products make life easier!

- DIY
- Consumer Electronics
- Crafts

- Software
- Cookware
- Hobbies

- Videos
- Music
- Games
- and More!

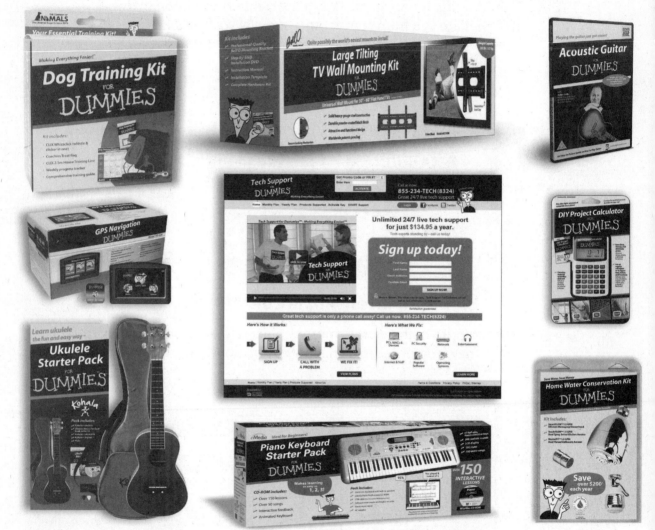

For more information, go to **Dummies.com** and search the store by category.

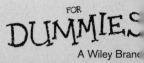

A Wiley Brand